MW01505619

Eat Your Way To Health:

Healing, Kindness & The Plant Life Cycle

Madhava Das

Transcendigital Productions

Published by Transendigital Productions
16251 Haleakala Hwy.
Kula, Maui, Hawaii 96790
808-878-6821

Legal Disclaimer: Nothing written in this book should be viewed as a substitute exclusive of competent medical care.

ISBN 978-0-9847258-9-2

Library of Congress Control Number: 2012930714

Printed in the U.S.A.

Contents

Eat Your Way To Health

Healing, Kindness & The Plant Life Cycle

Steps To Success

Preface:

Freedom

Heart disease, cancer, stroke, diabetes, Alzheimer's disease, multiple sclerosis, and so on, are all diseases that don't need to happen, or if they do happen to progress.

No animals need to be killed for humans to be perfectly healthy.

With a healthy and kind diet, good appearance is maintained, aging is slowed, and degenerative diseases are prevented, stopped or reversed.

What is that healthy diet?

That healthy diet is similar to the diet Bill Clinton has adopted to reverse his heart disease: a whole food, calorie normal, no oil, vegan plant-based diet – more simply and accurately called the **Plant Life Cycle Diet**.

There are several good books about stopping and reversing **particular diseases**, and what they all have in common is that they all propound diets that are intimately related to the **plant's life cycle**.

All good diets are based on historical **calorie normality, with high nutrient-to-calorie ratios from whole plant foods.** High nutrient-to-calorie ratios are directly related to the **plant's life cycle**.

What is the **life cycle** of the plant and how are the plant's reproductive life cycle stages related to human **health**? That's what will be revealed in this book.

A special note here is that many say one can "now and then" eat almost anything and still remain healthy - the problem with that is the same problem one has if they are trying to quit smoking cigarettes. ADDICTION!

No one can quit smoking by "now and then" having a cigarette, or by smoking in "moderation".

"Now and then", and "moderation" in eating are marketing inspired inaccuracies. Moderate eating yields a moderate heart attack and a moderately early death. Healthy eating is like a balance scale – one drop too much on the wrong side and **over time** the scale tips way down.

Chapter 1
Plant Life Cycle Diet

We begin the chapters of the book with three quotes, and end the book with one:

"Nothing will benefit human health and increase chances for survival of life on Earth as much as the evolution to a vegetarian diet."

~ Albert Einstein

"A man can live and be healthy without killing animals for food; therefore, if he eats meat, he participates in taking animal life merely for the sake of his appetite."

~ Leo Tolstoy, author of War And Peace.

"It ill becomes us to invoke in our daily prayers the blessings of God, the Compassionate, if we in turn will not practice elementary compassion towards our fellow creatures."

~ Mahatma Gandhi

The Greek mathematician Pythagoras was an ethical or "kindness" vegetarian, and vegetarians were often called Pythagoreans until the vegetarian word was created in the mid 1800's.

Socrates was a disciple of Pythagoras, and Plato was a disciple of Socrates. All were ethical vegetarians.

Today many young people are going the kindness route also.

But what about health? Isn't abstention from eating meat dangerous for health?

No - on the contrary, modern science has revealed that the diet of disease REVERSAL & PREVENTION, and of ANTI-AGING - is guess what?…

… a calorie normal, whole food/no oil, plant-based diet - more insightfully called the **PLANT LIFE CYCLE DIET**.

The independent work of Doctors Castelli, Campbell, Roberts, & many others have shown that **as the best markers**, if you keep your total blood cholesterol number below 150 mg/dL & your LDL below 80 by natural means, not by drugs, you become cardiovascular DISEASE- **PROOF**.

Inflammation is the culprit. When total & LDL cholesterol are very low all the other things you've heard about cholesterol details are moot points and are simply academic investigations.

More importantly, calorie restriction (CR) - studied since 1935 - is the ONLY intervention that has established that **at any age**, by reducing calorie intake while maintaining or increasing total aggregate nutrients you may **SIGNIFICANTLY** decrease **all** degenerative diseases, and **SIGNIFICANTLY increase <u>vigorous fully cognizant lifespan</u>**.

Be advised that **vested interests** have, however, consciously and/or unconsciously distorted what they call <u>calorie restriction</u> (& almost anything else you can think of in the way of healthy eating).

In studies of mammals and of other species - one group of subjects are allowed to eat all they want in a laboratory environment while other groups are given various lesser percentages of the amount of food eaten by the unrestricted group.

In a natural environment, including humans in evolutionary pre-industrial times, the environment naturally and automatically limited maximum food intake (droughts, floods, other animals, et cetera) and no one ate the amounts of food that unrestricted lab subjects and the average Joe eat in modern times.

In other words modern unrestricted subjects are eating a gluttonous diet and the so-called "restricted" subjects are eating an evolutionarily **NORMAL** amount of calories.

With profits in mind, today's vested interests consciously or unconsciously want you to continue being gluttons, and are trying to scare you by calling a calorie normal (CN) diet with high natural nutrients – they are calling that evolutionarily normal diet – "starvation" or "restriction".

Calorie normality without nutrient restriction (CN) is **not** starvation or restriction - but is the totally **normal** pattern humans have been quite **happy** and **prosperous** with for **thousands** and **thousands** of years. I'll repeat this statement later in the book.

Calorie restriction [actually calorie normality with high nutrients] is the ONLY way proven to significantly extend healthy life span (up to 60%) in virtually all species tested from amoeba, to snail, to spider, to cow, fish, horse, dog, cat, monkey and by way of aging markers to humans. No other intervention can match the proven results of CR/CN with high nutrients. Not by exercising, not by taking vitamins, not by taking food supplements et cetera.

To quote the National Institute on Aging, National Institutes of Health (NIH) – January 2007:

"Dietary caloric restriction [calorie normality with high nutrients] **is the only intervention repeatedly demonstrated to retard the**

onset and incidence of age-related diseases, maintain function, and extend both lifespan and health span in mammals, including brain and behavioral function."

See abstract of study and photos at:
http://www.MadhavaDas.com/primate.gif
http://www.MadhavaDas.com/primates.gif
This is very important, please do this now.

Keeping your total cholesterol below 150 and LDL below 80 eliminates heart disease - and CR/CN is champ in increasing **all-disease-free, fully cognizant lifespan.** CR/CN and achieving truly low cholesterol numbers - it turns out - are both related to the **plant's life cycle**.

Universal Misconception

An almost universal misconception/distortion about how to determine which foods have the highest nutrient levels is helping to cause untold confusion about proper diet. Marketing sometimes distorts things.

Nutrients are almost universally reported **per gram**-weight or per serving, which is **HIGHLY MISLEADING** in light of calorie restriction studies.

CR/CN studies, without controversy, have shown that the accurate view is that of a **PER CALORIE** DETERMINATION OF NUTRIENTS – NOT PER GRAM.

The difference between per gram (or per serving), and per calorie may seem small, but is actually on the order of the difference between a flat earth and the earth as it is.

You may gain the advantages of a so-called calorie restricted - but actually a calorie normal diet, **WITHOUT HUNGER** by eating foods with the highest nutrients per <u>calorie</u> density, which may be termed calorie efficient foods. **Nutrients per calorie density follows the plant's reproductive life cycle**, with the first structure, the leaf, being the highest.

Calorie efficient foods are by nature's arrangement also **high volume foods and easily fill your stomach** without excess calories. **Efficiency, in all ways, follows the plant's life cycle**.

It turns out that the highest nutrient-per-calorie foods are also the foods that allow total cholesterol & LDL to easily stay below disease proof 150 and 80 levels respectively.

Throughout evolutionary history we ate <u>mostly</u> vegetables and fruits - and what may seem like calorie restriction in light of today's super-abundance of high calorie foods is really CALORIE NORMALITY WITH HIGH NUTRIENTS.

Calorie efficient foods provide you with the healthiest, disease preventative diet possible. But rest assured - <u>taste is not restricted</u> in this diet!

Knowing both the science of calorie efficient foods, and the real attainable results of the **Plant Life Cycle Diet** is highly motivational to people of all ages. Seniors, juniors, business people, administrators, workers, educators, students and people in general will all benefit to receive this knowledge.

King Ashoka, Copernicus And Bill Clinton

In ancient times King Ashoka of India adopted and thereby helped spread Buddhism.

Former president Bill Clinton has adopted a calorie normal **plant life cycle vegan diet,** that when faithfully followed, lowers your blood cholesterol into the degenerative-disease-proof range AND extends cognizant, vital lifespan via calorie normality with high nutrients.

Just like Copernicus revolutionalized our position in the universe - **plant-sourced, plant life cycle based nutrition may be about to revolutionize our eating habits and health.**

Bill Clinton's adoption of a **healthy** vegan diet may signal the Copernican phyto-centric coming of age of plant-sourced nutrition - the **Plant Life Cycle Diet**.

Copernicus knew the reaction his discovery would have, and so he delayed publishing his book until he was more or less on his deathbed. It took 100 years after his death until his idea was accepted as fact.

Let us hope that the disease reversing diet Bill Clinton has adopted becomes accepted well before 100 years and millions of unnecessary early deaths have occurred.

The main idea in <u>healthy</u> eating is of **highest nutrient-to-calorie ratio foods**. It's not so much, for example, that there is something wrong with fat per se, other than the fact that fat has more than twice the calories per bite as carbohydrates and protein, and thus fat has about half the nutrient to calorie ratio. Separated out - oil is almost astronomically calorie rich & nutrient poor – and deadly. As you shall see later in this book.

Whole plant foods are potent because they are much lower in calories and have higher nutrient to calorie ratios than both animal products and processed / fractionated plant foods like oil, sugar, white flower & white rice, including dried fruit and fruit juice.

Because of the combination of **SUPER AVAILABILITY AND ADDICTION - high-calorie <u>whole</u> plant foods** like avocados, olives, nuts, and coconut (but not coconut water) and also calorie concentrated foods like dried fruit and fruit juice, also need to be watched or possibly eliminated to have your total cholesterol stay down below the 150 mg/dL disease proof, CR/CN life extending level. **DIET MANAGEMENT TO CONTROLL BLOOD CHOLESTEROL LEVELS IS THE KEY!!!**

Calorie heaviness goes up as the plant's **growing life cycle** progresses, then continues up more - beyond the disease proof level, starting with both processed plant foods and all animal products. The young leaf is best, followed by older leaves, buds, flowers, vegetable-fruits, fresh fruits, tubers & roots, and legumes. More borderline but acceptable are whole grains. High taste seed spices as flavorings, are great in small amounts.

Health Mantra

We have all heard the mantra: "Eat more fruits and vegetables."

According to virtually every major health organization in the United States - like the **American Heart Association, American Cancer Society, Alzheimer's Association, American Diabetes Association et cetera, and the United Nation's World Health Organization (WHO)** - we should, "Eat more fruits and vegetables."

They all are wrong. We should **NOT** "Eat more fruits and vegetables."

Wrong Way Corrigan

Everyone knows, "Eat more fruits and vegetables." But that is wrong.

Better but not best is: "Eat more *vegetables & fruits*."

Green leafy vegetables and other starch-less vegetable-fruits **come before** sweet fruits and all other categories of foods. More on this momentarily.

Not only is the order of vegetables and fruits reversed, but the: "Eat more" part is also wrong.

Many of us are overweight. So if we only "eat more" of anything, what's going to happen? Duh!

Should be: **Eat Only Whole Plant Parts, Including Plenty Of Greens, Vegetable-Fruits & Fruits: ~And Zero Processed & Animal Products~**

Green Vegetables

Green leafy vegetables as a staple, with other vegetable-fruits, buds (like broccoli), berries & fruits also as staples, along with tubers and roots (like sweet potatoes), legumes, grains & seeds, a variety of spices, and if you don't take iodized salt then iodine from various sea vegetables, and a methylcobalamin vitamin B12 supplement (and if desired, B12 additionally from a good nutritional yeast) - is very close to the perfect diet. Oh… plus sunshine and a little exercise.

Beans, whole grains, seeds and nuts are more calorie dense and therefore **more & more addictive in that order**, and for weight-loss can be minimized. Their <u>excessive</u> consumption is encouraged only on major holidays, and at parties, and weddings - ha, ha. No… seriously.

A diet without beans and seeds would not really be a diet without beans and seeds.

OK - you have 10 seconds to figure that one out. Tic, tic, tic…

What do fruits contain?

Duh, seeds! For example green beans have little beans in them, snap peas have little peas in them, tomatoes, cucumbers, eggplants, okras etc. – all are full of seeds that we eat along with the fruits.

Those immature seeds have a high percentage of water in them and are in limited amount compared to the fruit, and therefore are not effective in trying to push your body's PH balance to the harmful acid inflammatory side. More on acid/alkaline later.

Nuts contain significant amounts of **saturated** fat, and most are high in omega-**6** fatty acids (the 1st number of each number pair in the following <u>e</u>ssential <u>f</u>atty <u>a</u>cid EFA Ratios chart – the second numbers are omega-3's). High omega-6 to omega-3 ratios are inflammatory and unhealthy. If you are going to eat a few nuts, walnuts have the best omega-6 to omega-3 ratio.

Here are Jeff Novick's (MS, RD, LD, LN) charts on the subject.

Percent Saturated Fat Of Nuts/Seeds

◆ Black Walnuts	5%	◆ Brazil Nut	21%
◆ English Walnuts	8%	◆ Almonds	6%
◆ Pecans	8%	◆ Pumpkin Seeds	14%
◆ Pistachio	8.5%	◆ Sunflower Seeds	6.5%
◆ Pine Nuts	6.6%	◆ CA Avocados	11.5%
◆ Macadamia	15%	◆ FL Avocados	15%
◆ Hazelnut	6.5%	◆ Flaxseed	6%
◆ Cashew	12.5%	◆ Chia Seed	6%

Jeff Novick

EFA Ratios Of Nuts/Seeds

◆ Black Walnuts	16:1	◆ Brazil Nut	1000:1
◆ English Walnuts	4:1	◆ Almonds	1800:1
◆ Pecans	20:1	◆ Pumpkin Seeds	117:1
◆ Pistachio	37:1	◆ Sunflower Seeds	300:1
◆ Pine Nuts	300:1	◆ CA Avocados	15:1
◆ Macadamia	6:1	◆ FL Avocados	16.5:1
◆ Hazelnut	88:1	◆ Flaxseed	3.9:1
◆ Cashew	117:1	◆ Chia Seed	3:1

Jeff Novick

Plant Life Cycle Diet

Nutrient density - **compared** to **calories** - is what is important, and nutrient density follows the order of the plant's growing life cycle.

It turns out that most all nutrients appear and are created in leaves of plants. Green leafy vegetables are HIGHEST in nutrients and LOWEST in calories.

Green leafy vegetables and some solid green vegetables including things like **broccoli** (a flower bud related to a leaf) have the **highest nutrients to calorie ratio**. Green leafy vegetables have the highest overall nutrient density and are the **healthiest** foods - **by far**.

Green leafy vegetables and some solid bud-vegetables including things like **broccoli** & **cauliflower** and various vegetable-fruits should be our **STAPLE** foods - UNLESS YOU ARE **VERY** POOR and live in a third world country - then legumes and whole grains are a more economical source of calories. OR unless you are a full time athlete or heavy construction worker, then you could eat a lot of vegetables AND a lot of roots & tubers like sweet potatoes, and some legumes.

When a seed **sprouts**, the tender green leaf is at the very highest point of aggregate nutrients per calorie density.

Mature but tender **leafy vegetable**s are a natural **staple** food. And they grow to harvest the quickest.

In **prehistoric evolutionary** times, humans originated and lived in tropical and sub-tropical regions and this is what people ate – mostly easily available (they don't run away from you) green leaf vegetables, vegetable-fruits including legume-fruits (like green beans), and berries & other fruits.

The next stage in the **life cycle of a plant** as it matures and grows after the appearance of leaves, is the appearance of flower buds and flowers. Broccoli is in this category. Flower petals are specialized types of leaves.

Next to form in a **plant's life cycle** after the flower, is the fruit. Here anti-oxidants are high and calories begin to concentrate a bit, therefore, from the nutrient density standpoint, fruits (especially sweet fruits) are generally a little less desirable than leafy greens and edible buds & flowers.

As a plant grows, the sooner an above-ground part of a plant appears in the <u>plant's reproductive life cycle</u>, the higher it's aggregate nutrients per <u>calorie</u> ratio and the healthier that plant part is for you to eat.

Just below you see photos of the parts of a plant in the order they appear in the <u>plants' life cycle</u>.

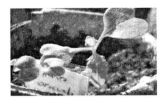

Sprouted Leaf – (Kale)

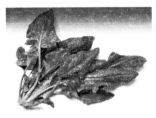

Mature Leaf – (Spinach)

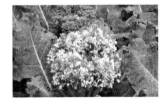

Flower (bud)– (Broccoli)

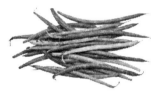

Fruit – (Green Bean)

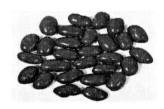

Seed – (Kidney Bean)

After the leaf, bud / flower, and fruit comes the seed – beans, grains, seeds & nuts are very concentrated energy. Seeds & nuts have high **calorie** density - not good in high quantities if you have trouble maintaining a low weight.

Generally the leaf is the healthiest food, followed by the bud / flower, then the fruit, then the root / tuber – this is where the root / tuber fits in.

Most of the so-called roots we eat are actually specialized underground food storage **stem-tubers** – the potato for example, or **root-tubers** – sweet potatoes, or are even balls of specialized underground **leaves** – the onion.

Going back above ground - after the fruit develops the seed develops.

From leaf, to flower, to fruit, to tuber, to seed - that's the order of increasing heaviness. That's the order of buying choice, the order of eating choice, etc - and the order of disease prevention.

Legumes to some extent, and grains especially can be minimized but not necessarily eliminated - except unlimited use is encouraged on special occasions like weddings & holiday feasts. Hooray!

The best health mantra is: "Give me something green." This is **Plant Life Cycle Nutrition**, or the **Plant Life Cycle Diet**.

A plant's own worldly purpose is to collect energy to ensure it reproduces its genes. The leaf is the collecting agent.

Underground root-tubers, roots and stem-tubers, and underground **leaf** bulbs are storage vessels of collected energy - as are seeds.

Alkaline reacting root-tubers, roots and stem-tubers are different than beans and grain, as they don't cause a negative <u>inflammatory</u> acid response in the body like beans and grains. Tubers are the better calorie source.

The order of heaviness from lightest to heaviest is: leaves, buds/flowers, vegetable-fruits, sweet fruits, then underground energy storage parts and then seeds - the **plant life cycle**.

Animal foods are generally more calorie heavy and don't have any or much of many various anti-oxidants – or fiber, but do have very many degenerative disease causing properties.

Tubers and roots although energy storage plant parts - are a little less calorie dense than beans, grains, seeds and nuts (by the way, all seeds contain a complete baby plant embryo). Again, tubers and roots are not acid forming like beans and grains.

A note of caution: There are differences between various website lists of what specific foods are acid forming and what are alkaline. But again, beans and grains are acid forming - tubers are not.

From leaf, to flower, to fruit, to tuber & root, to legume (inclusion of legumes will be explained in Chapter 6) – all these foods are very healthy. Grains and nuts are more borderline for various reasons.

There are "pro" and "cautious" groups in plant-based nutrition as far as nuts are concerned. The harmonizing view comes from a good understanding of calorie restriction / calorie normality.

As briefly alluded to before, there is nothing wrong with healthy fat per se. The problem is excess calorie-density - caused by the fact that fat is more than two times more calorie dense than carbs or protein.

If you can maintain low weight and low blood cholesterol levels (below 150 total & 80 LDL) while eating a few nuts that's great – if not then don't eat nuts. It's pretty simple.

GO BY YOUR OWN PERSONAL LAB CHOLESTEROL TEST RESULTS – NOT BY WHAT ONE GROUP OR ANOTHER SAYS!

It cannot be stressed enough how important it is to **know and control your total and LDL blood cholesterol levels**. **150** and **80** mg/dL respectively are the **SIMPLE MEASURABLE MARKERS !!!** that tell you if you are going to die early due to degenerative disease.

They are like the altimeter and airspeed indicator in an airplane – **IF YOU DON'T KNOW YOUR NUMBERS, YOU'RE GOING TO CRASH.**

If you keep your numbers pegged below 150 and 80 you'll soar like a bird.

You will hear all kinds of things out there about cholesterol levels and there is some truth there. BUT that is about what goes on at high cholesterol levels way above the degenerative disease proof level.

Levels below 150 mg/dL total and 80 mg/dL LDL are virtually magical. All the complications of high blood fat go away.

Calorie Normal Plant Life Cycle Diet

The younger the plant part you eat, the younger and healthier you stay.

The calorie normal **Plant Life Cycle Diet** is at once the new revolutionary diet and lifestyle we have all been searching for, and the oldest original diet of both Bhagavad-Gita and Genesis. Both East & West.

If for any reason you desire to be healthy and live a long life, the Eat Your Way To Health - **Plant Life Cycle Diet** is for you. With an open mind, after finishing this book all confusion about diet will be cleared up and you will have an understanding of the ideal diet. Whether you act on your new knowledge or not is your decision.

This book is being written as an offering of my experience and knowledge for the purpose of giving back to help others.

If you find any errors of science in this book, please send an email to: mdasNow@gmail.com, and it will be investigated and corrected as necessary.

In the just concluded Chapter 1 you heard about calorie normality, nutrient density, the plant's life cycle and the **Plant Life Cycle Diet**. After a brief recounting of my particular journey in the following Chapter 2, Chapter 3 explains more nutrient per calorie details of the calorie normal **Plant Life Cycle Diet** with a list of all the specifics of the diet. Chapters 4 through 7 give the scientifically established evidence-based details. Chapter 8 is titled: The Flavors of India. Chapter 9 gives additional information - and more.

Chapter 2
Few Challenges Left

After being discharged from the U.S. Air Force at the end of the Vietnam War, I helped found the United States Hang Gliding Association and in 1972 successfully completed the first hot air balloon drop of a hang glider east of the Rockies thousands of feet directly over the intersection of two interstate highways in Central Pennsylvania.

Around that same time I contributed to the design of the first successful human powered aircraft, the Gossamer Condor now hanging at the Smithsonian Air & Space Museum in Washington D.C. beside the original Wright Brothers flyer and the Apollo 11 command module that took the first humans to walk on the moon.

I say these things not to boast, (oh, well, maybe a little) but to establish leading edge action and scientific thought.

I had been living a life of luxury at Hermosa Beach in Southern California - traveling back and forth coast-to-coast eating steak and eggs for breakfast. I thought the full-length two-tone black and brown leather coat I would wear over my white T-shirt and blue jeans was the epitome of Hollywood cool.

But I was headed for hell.

A friend noticed my chronic deep, really deep chest cough – I was coughing up thick lung mucus - and gave me professor Arnold Ehret's Mucusless Diet Healing System Lessen Course completed in 1922 which says green and starch-less vegetables and fruits are mucus-less foods.

One-day while flying in my hang glider I misjudged the distance to the landing zone, hit the top of a tall tree and fell 40 feet to what should have been my certain death.

One month later after being released from the hospital and at the philosophy and religion section of the local bookstore I found a book - Beyond Birth and Death - the author A.C. Bhakivedanta, who was from India, followed a diet of milk and plant-based foods.

I knew Indian civilization had survived for thousands of years on a milk and plant based diet. So it was Ehret's fruits and vegetables - with milk as insurance.

That was in 1976. Fast forward to 2003 when in a month's time I heard about the latest science on omega-3 fats and vitamin B12, and heard Gene Baur speak about and saw his video, Life Behind Bars detailing cruelty to farm and dairy animals on industrial factory farms.

http://en.wikipedia.org/wiki/Gene_Baur

I changed my eating habits for health, ethical and spiritual reasons, and because my mother died from cancer less than a year after retiring from having taught mostly first and second graders for over forty years.

Whatever motivation drives your interest in health, beauty, kindness and longevity, may all human beings live a full century in vibrant, cognizant, compassionate health - a real possibility with the scientifically, ethically and spiritually bona fide Eat Your Way To Health, Calorie Normal, **Plant Life Cycle Diet**.

Chapter 3
Nutrient Per Calorie Descent

As mentioned before, there is only one way that's proven experimentally in virtually all tested animal species including amoebas, worms, slugs, spiders, mice, rats, guinea pigs, fish, dogs, cows and preliminarily in both rhesus & squirrel monkeys - and now in human beings in the form of verified health and aging markers - to **significantly** extend average and maximum **vigorous** life span. And to correspondingly delay onset of degenerative diseases such as heart attack, cancer, stroke, osteoporosis, diabetes, Alzheimer's (which has undergone a twelve fold increase in the past twenty years) etc.

No other intervention has been shown to significantly extend healthy cognizant life span.

That one way is to reduce the number of calories in the diet while maintaining a high nutrient level.

Again this is the same diet that has been demonstrated to **STOP AND REVERSE** cardio-vascular disease - the numero uno devotee of the grim reaper.

In human beings, **calorie normality** with high nutrients (CN) may easily be done without being hungry by eating the highest aggregate nutrients per calorie foods.

Again, it is VERY important to note that this is nutrients per calorie, NOT nutrients per gram or per serving. The body **gains weight**, **ages**, and **gets diseased** according to calories, not according to grams!

Per gram calculations of which foods to eat are as misleading in the modern age as flat-earth calculations of orbits and trajectories would be in this age of satellites and rockets to the stars.

Look at this chart to see the distortion.

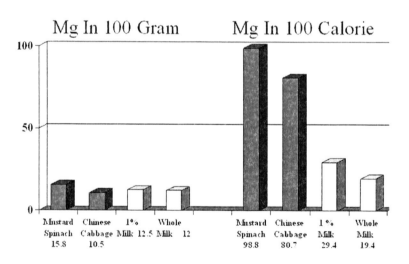

Calcium Comparison

Advertising by the dairy industry has distorted our perception of the comparative calcium level of milk - to make us think milk is far superior to anything else, when if fact milk is far **inferior** to greens as we see here.

All this started out innocently years ago but in light of modern scientific measurement and insight, the dairy industries (among many other food manufacturers) are straight out liars.

The very **UN**FORTUNATE situation at present is that almost universally, nutrients are thought of and reported according to the misleading nutrient per gram idea or per serving size – instead of per calorie.

Easily reducing the number of calories in the human diet while maintaining the same nutrient level - the key to health, weight loss and longevity - is possible because we now know by scientific analysis what are the highest nutrient per calorie foods...

THEY FOLLOW THE PLANT'S LIFE CYCLE.

Below is a very important bar chart showing the descending aggregate nutrients per calorie **continuum or hierarchy**.

Green leafy vegetables - the highest category, are indexed at a positive value of 100.

Per calorie, and per gram information from the USDA on 26 different nutrients (including protein, vitamins, lipids et cetera for most whole unprocessed foods and too many processed junk foods) is available at:

http://www.MadhavaDas.com/n_database.xls
[Note: Large file with long download time.]

Here is the very revealing and important chart:

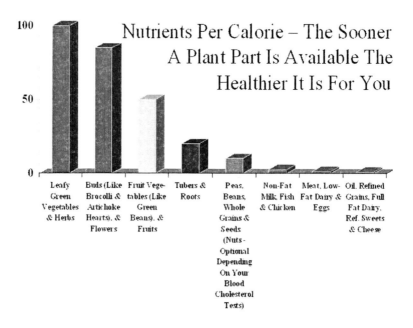

Nutrient density per calorie occurs on a **continuum or in a hierarchy** going downward from the leaf. In other words - leafy vegetables have the highest total nutrient density per calorie.

Note: The chart is subject to relatively minor adjustments because rating total aggregate nutrient density has several slightly differing statistical formulas, and because there may be – as in many things - exceptions to the rule.

But the chart is quite sufficient for showing the **big** picture of the **continuum or hierarchy** of nutrient density per **calorie**, not per gram. PER CALORIE NUTRIENT DENSITY **DESCENDS** AND FOLLOWS CLOSELY, FOR ALL PRACTICAL PURPOSES, THE REPRODUCTIVE **LIFE CYCLE OF THE PLANT**.

The old idea of **"food groups"** is like the idea that the earth is flat. Traditional food groups is a false idea and is outdated, and is dangerous and misleading – so of course vested interests use the outdated idea of food groups to mislead you, confuse you and bamboozle you. More on this later.

This is irresponsible on their part and borders on criminal - as do the quotes "find the right balance" and "all things in moderation". If it's bad - **zero** is the right amount.

Like cigarettes or atomic bombs ... zero.

And now some specifics on the diet:

The **Plant Life Cycle Diet** consists of:

1) Raw and cooked green leaf, and solid bud-vegetables like broccoli, and green leaf herbs such as basil, mint, parsley, sage, rosemary and thyme.

2) Plenty of colorful vegetable-fruits, berries & sweet fruits.

3) Lesser amounts of tubers & roots, and legumes.

4) Lesser amounts of whole grains (acid forming & tends to leaches calcium along with other problems). **No processed oil.** If your total cholesterol is below 150 mg/dL and LDL below 80 nuts headed by walnuts. Test nuts yourself by having "with" & "without" blood tests.

5) Omega-3 is in green leafy vegetables, including purslane. Get vitamin B12 in tablet form and/or via high nutrient per calorie, high vitamin B12 **nutritional yeast**. Have your level of B12 tested when you get your cholesterol tested and adjust accordingly. For example, taking 1,000 mcg weekly my B12 level was above the upper limit of the reference range so I cut down to 2,000 mcg once per month.

With a varied and purified diet and getting sufficient sunlight, except for B12 no other supplement is normally needed. More on B12 in Chapter 7.

Please just think that the Perfect Diet **emphasizes**: green vegetables and other vegetables, with berries, fruits, tubers & roots, and with some legumes. I prefer to use whole grains **as side dishes** - and only occasionally as main dishes.

On **holidays and feast occasions** prepare and eat all the grain **main-dish** preparations you like. In other words you may want to think of **large main-dish grain preparations, and preparations containing lots of nuts** as special major holiday feast and wedding et cetera **CELEBRATION** items.

Try to eat the various plant parts in the order and proportions according to the size of the bars in the Nutrients Per Calorie Continuum chart on previous and forthcoming pages. You'll get some more info on portion sizes a few pages from now.

Virtually everyone agrees that greens are our best nutritious food. I'll make an educated guess & say people who live the very longest are probably salad eaters.

Broccoli - a flower bud - has some fame as a good food. Most everyone loves a sweet piece of fruit on a hot summer day. Foliage, flowers and fruits.

The diet of primates. The diet of Genesis. The diet of ahimsa Buddhists. The diet of Bhagavad-Gita. The Eat Your Way To Health, **Plant Life Cycle,** Whole, Calorie Normal, No-Added-Oil **Die**t.

Specifically, in simple form here's what to eat in order from best (leaves at the top) - to acceptable (whole grains and seed spices at the bottom):

Calorie normal, whole plant parts in life cycle growing order:

- Leaves, stems, buds & flowers
- Vegetable-fruits including legume fruits, berries and sweet fruits
- Tubers and roots - especially sweet potatoes
- Legumes
- Whole grains; and a small amount of high taste seeds as flavorings.

And not to eat:

Animal derived foods:

- No meat, fish, eggs, poultry, or dairy including skim milk and yogurt.

Processed plant foods:

- Oil in any form (including olive oil), or as an ingredient in any food – zero!
- No vegetable milks like soymilk, rice milk, nut milks, etc. as they contain added oil and processed gum ingredients and/or are just generally too rich.

- No bread that contains <u>oil or any other processed ingredients</u>, even so-called 100% whole wheat bread — **unless** you can find or make your own 100% whole wheat bread with <u>zero oil and **ZERO** processed ingredients</u>.
- Sugar in any form including dried sugar cane juice, corn syrup & Sucanat, all of which are too calorie dense.
- Tofu – processed and mostly fat.

Calorie dense whole plant foods to be eaten only if your total cholesterol stays below 150 mg/dL & LDL below 80:

- Nuts & non-spice seeds – are very rich. Despite their nutrients they are high calorie.
- Avocados – ditto.
- Olives – ditto.
- Coconut & coconut milk, but coconut water is ok.

****

A Large Amount Of Greens Is Calorie Equal To A Small Amount Of Beans

That was the list of what to eat, and what not to eat.

Now <u>how much</u> of each good thing to eat?

You will be eating a <u>large</u> volume of greens, broccoli, vegetable-fruits & sweet fruits – a smaller volume of tubers, and legumes, & also a small volume of grains & seeds. **When you do this you are getting approximately EQUAL calories from each type of plant part.** Remember that plant-parts are less desirable and more **calorie dense** as the plant's life cycle progresses, i.e. as the plant gets older and has more time to collect more energy / calories.

Below are photos, thanks to WiseGeek.com, of 200-calorie portions of a few different plant parts that I have cut in half to 100-calorie portions. They used 200-calorie portions because they thought the bean and grain portions would look too small.

The pictured hundred-calorie portions are about right and the photos are in order of the plant's life cycle.

They didn't have photos of some other things like greens, vegetable-fruits and/or sweet potatoes. I wish they had. But you can see how from top to bottom the portions form a rough funnel shape. A note being that sweet potatoes are about 1½ x more calorie dense than carrots and would be a smaller volume than the carrots pictured.

Here are 100-calorie portions in life cycle order, showing decrease in volume but **equality** in calories:

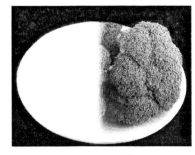

Broccoli – A Bud 100 calories

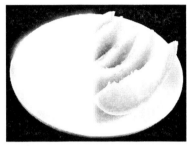

Honeydew – A Fruit 100 cal.

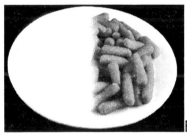

Baby Carrots – A Root 100c.
Sweet Potatoes Are Smaller

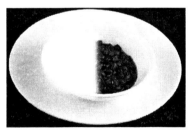

Black Beans – Beans 100 c.

So by eating a large (but not unlimited) volume of leaves, buds, stems, vegetable-fruits, and sweet fruits; a smaller volume of tubers like sweet potatoes, and of beans; and a small amount of grains and spice seeds, you will be getting a **calorie balanced, historically calorie-normal** diet with high nutrients (only from the recent modern gluttonous perspective would it be called a calorie restricted diet). This is a quite normal diet.

And thereby live a long **disease-free, cruelty-free** life.

Lab Test Results

On July 26, 2010, I had my blood tested. I had been eating oil and nuts but not animal products - my total cholesterol was lab tested to be 229, and LDL 146. Both bad.

On August 17, 2010, just 3 weeks later, my lab-tested results were: total cholesterol 127 and LDL 69.

What are the cardiovascular disease proof levels?

150 total and 80 LDL. What are my new numbers? …127 total and 69 LDL.

How'd I do it? The only change in my vegan diet was … no oil & no nuts, and more or less no sugar or dried fruits. (I'm not perfect; I think I ate a few raisins.)

If I had been eating animal products, my numbers would have been higher in the first test, and like my father and grandfather who each died of a heart attack, I'd probably be dead and not writing this book.

There is a discussion in healthy eating circles - to eat nuts, or not to eat nuts.

Just prior to the July test I had been reading the pro-nut literature and was influenced to eat nuts. And although I knew not to eat oil – I was still eating oil.

When I saw the 229 number I decided I really had to stop with the oil and nuts. So I did - and the results are life saving to say the least.

To further test things, I added back to my diet the small amount of nuts recommended, while continuing zero oil.

I then had another test done, and my total cholesterol rose to 175, a level drugs-and-surgery medicine would say is great - but still well above the cardio-vascular disease PROOF level of 150. **You may be different and can eat nuts** – I can't. Test nut intake on yourself with a pair of blood cholesterol tests.

I have absolutely no desire or craving to eat oil, or animal products ever again, and if you follow the recommendations, and thereby see your cholesterol numbers drop in three weeks down into the disease proof zone - you won't either.

Here's my highlighted before and after, lab print-outs – going from a cholesterol of 229 to 127 in 22 days:

Eat Your Way To Health

Honolulu, HI

---- CBC PROFILE ----

			Reference			
BLOOD	07/26 2010 11:01		Units	Ranges		

SERUM	CHOL	TRIG	HDL	LDLCAL
Ref range low	0		35	0
Ref range high	200	149		130
	mg/dL	mg/dL	mg/dL	mg/dL

----

a 07/26/2010 11:01   229 H   239 H 35.2   146 H
  a. Evaluation for CHOL:
     LOW RISK   = <200   mg/dL
     BORDERLINE RISK= 201-239 mg/dL
     HIGH RISK   = >240   mg/dL
     Evaluation for TRIG:
     New Reference Range effective 07/02/09
     NORMAL   = <150   mg/dL
     BORDERLINE HIGH = 150 -199   mg/dL
     HIGH   = 200 -499   mg/dL
     VERY HIGH   = >=500   mg/dL
     Evaluation for HDL:
     NORMAL = >35 md/dL

Report from: NEW MEXICO

Report Released Date/Time:
Provider: ADAY,DAVID B
  Specimen: BLOOD.   HEME 0818 254
    Specimen Collection Date: 08/17/2010 23:00

CHOLESTEROL		127	mg/dL	Ref: <=200
Eval:	Reference Range:	Desirable:	<200 mg/dL	
Eval:		Borderline High:	200-239 mg/dL	
Eval:		High:	> or = 240 mg/dL	
TRIGLYCERIDE		111	mg/dL	Ref: <=150
Eval:	Normal Triglycerides:	<150	mg/dL	
Eval:	Borderline High:	150-199	mg/dL	
Eval:	High Triglyceride:	200-499	mg/dL	
Eval:	Very High Triglyceride:	> or = 500 mg/dL		
LDL-CHOL Calculation		69	mg/dL	Ref: <=130
Eval:	Reference range:			
Eval:	Optimal:	<100	mg/dL	
Eval:	Near to Optimal:	100-129 mg/dL		
Eval:	Borderline high:	130-159 mg/dL		
Eval:	High:	160-189 mg/dL		
Eval:	Very High:	> or = 190	mg/dL	

Problems With Animal Protein

Knowledge of cell damage caused by eating animal protein is less well known in the general population than is the knowledge of the damage caused by eating animal fat.

The Cornell-Oxford-China Project is the "Grand Prix" of all health and disease studies. In that study the damage inflicted by consumption of animal protein is revealed in great detail.

Dr. Dean Edell, self-proclaimed "America's Doctor", on national radio reported one of many relatively recent studies that determined that animal product consumption for example, increased the risk for prostate cancer in men.

Dr. Edell reported, "The strongest risk factor for prostate cancer mortality was animal products, such as meat and dairy products."

Dr. Edell ended the piece with the quote: "These results should provide guidance for reducing the risk of prostate and other cancers."

Backing up the findings of the Cornell-Oxford-China Project and Dr. Edell's report - Doctor Esselstyn has shown in practice that eliminating all animal products and oil from your diet reverses heart disease. Another doctor has now also demonstrated **cancer** preventative changes via a whole food, calorie normal, plant life cycle diet.

The following chart shows, by extending one more column pair to the right, that a100% plant sourced diet **virtually eliminates** death from heart attack & cancer. Note: The chart is produced jointly by the NIH & WHO.

Unrefined Plant Food Consumption vs. The Killer Diseases

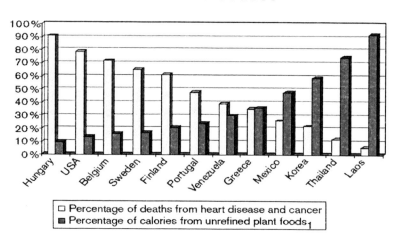

□ Percentage of deaths from heart disease and cancer
■ Percentage of calories from unrefined plant foods[1]

Combining the concept of calorie restriction (calorie normality) with the concept of high nutrient per **calorie foods** is **key** to understanding the calorie normal **Plant Life Cycle Diet 's** plant-based anti-aging, weight loss and degenerative disease preventing and reversing potency.

Scientific research is ongoing at the present time to explain in detail the particular mechanisms of the anti-aging of cells - or rather the premature aging of cells.

In simple terms we may understand that excess calories are inflammatory - in other words toxic.

Reducing calorie intake while maintaining or increasing nutrients - with all it's health & life extending benefits - without going hungry - is possible by eating high nutrient, high volume per calorie foods, and not eating high calorie junk & animal foods.

The best foods by far are the leafy and flower-bud vegetables - the towering pillars of the Plant Life Cycle Diet:

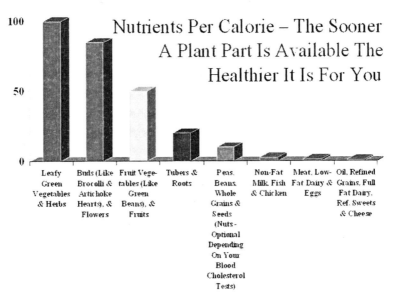

In various lists of nutrient density, according to slightly different ways of weighting and calculating individual importance of vitamins, minerals and phytochemicals; vegetables, both leafy and flower bud, and other vegetable-fruits and fruits always top the list.

After fruits some people say roots, some say beans. We don't argue the point too strongly, but in Chapter 5 we will talk about the significance of root crops replacing grains as far as maintaining **young-looking skin** - demonstrated by the residents of the village of Yuzuri Hara, Japan who have smooth unwrinkled skin well into advanced age.

The calorie normal **Plant Life Cycle Diet** is real, bona fide and available now. It is scientifically, spiritually and morally correct.

Don't accept the calorie normal **Plant Life Cycle Diet** because I say so - accept it because you want more out of life. The magic moment is when you make the decision and take the action to look younger and feel stronger.

By accepting the truth you will live in a higher plane. You will be the gainer; you will come into your normal position. The science is there. Scripture is there. Socrates is there.

You be there.

Chapter 4

Give Me Something Green

When my dear wife Sunanda, from India via Fiji, asks me what I want to eat for dinner... what do I say? "Give me something green."

If foods were money and leafy greens were hundred-dollar bills: each bud-vegetable could be worth about $90. Vegetable-fruits and sweet fruits might be $50 bills. Tubers and roots could be $18 to $20 bills.

Peas, beans, seeds and grains might range from about $15 down to say $6 bills. Nuts because of their high calories due to high fat content including saturated fat, and addictive properties, are more borderline.

Calorie restriction studies point to this.

The seed group is more borderline and in the gray area (that's why it's gray on the ebook's colored chart). Nuts contain saturated fat and most have high levels of Omega-6 fats and are discouraged, but are allowed in a cardiovascular disease preventing and reversing diet if your blood cholesterol levels stay below 150 total and 80 LDL.

Grains may be somewhat restricted in the **Plant Life Cycle Diet** not because they are high in carbohydrates or high in calories per se, but because they are borderline in nutrients per calorie, and have anti-nutrients.

The difference in nutrients per calorie between leaf, bud/flower, fruit and seed as **categories** is generally larger than the difference within each category.

That is to say **- it is less important to know which particular type of leafy green vegetable is best - than to know that overall leafy, and solid bud-vegetables (like broccoli, cauliflower and artichokes), and vegetable-fruits & sweet fruits are superior to other categories.**

It's not so important to worry about which fruit is better than the other, as it is to realize that fruits are somewhat less valuable than leafy, and solid bud-vegetables, but are higher than tubers and roots.

Which would you rather have a hundred-dollar bill, or a twenty-dollar bill? After that - we may be concerned with the highest nutrient foods within each of the plant-part categories: leaves, stems & buds; vegetable-fruits; sweet fruits; roots & tubers; and seeds.

Use the high (not the highest green leafy and bud vegetables) - use the high nutrient per calorie foods, i.e. vegetable-fruits, sweet fruits, tubers and roots, to complement the high protein, low calorie greens. Legumes especially – and grains are OK if you are not overweight and not sensitive to them.

About 35-40% of the calories in greens come from protein. Legumes around 25%. Tubers approximately 6.5 to 7%. Fruits are roughly 3% protein. In comparison human mother's milk is about 6% of calories from protein.

A combination of greens, lots of vegetable-fruits, fruits, some tubers, and a few legumes over the course of a day or two, naturally balance out to around the 9.5% of protein that primates as a group eat in nature.

Fruits are low in protein but high in anti-oxidants. Tubers and roots have more protein than the just mentioned 6% of human mother's milk.

Again, greens are the highest total nutrients per calorie foods - by far.

Meat, fish, eggs, butter, cheese, milk, yogurt, oil, sugar, and "refined" (Orwellian Newspeak for fractionated) processed foods, are chump change or worse and have negative effects.

Overweight But Undernourished

It is an understatement to say you may have heard that too many Americans are overweight including more and more young children. But we also often hear the following quote or something like it: "Feed the hungry, feed the hungry. We should feed our own starving children before giving aid to foreign countries!" Politics aside, which is it - are we overfed or underfed?

Mostly overfed, but undernourished.

In a wealthy country it needn't be that way.

Part of the problem is that to stay ahead of the competition, food-processing companies have to always keep inventing new processed foods.

Walk down the isle in a supermarket's breakfast cereal or snack food section… duh.

The meat, fish and dairy industries are BIG advertisers.

Way back in 1989 for example McDonald's Corporation spent over one million dollars per day advertising its products. How'd you like to have one day's worth of McDonald's add-budget handed to you?

Another problem and **perhaps the biggest** is tradition / culture / relatives. "Thanksgiving is Thursday." "The Fourth of July is Saturday." "Christmas is coming soon." **It takes a strongly motivated individual to break free of their political history and religious dietary traditions.**

Are you strongly motivated?

It is so important to have support when trying to change eating habits.

For example, in the October 1998 issue of Health Education & Behavior, Gloria Sorensen, PhD, MPH, of the Dana-Farber Cancer Institute in Boston reported from a study of more than 1,300 health care workers by the **National Cancer Institute** that workers in a program to increase their intake of fruits and vegetables are more likely to change their diet if they have strong support from co-workers and family members.

Through studies of Seventh Day Adventists we know that average vegetarian diets over a lifetime yield a five- to 10-year lengthening of life. This is done even without attempting calorie restriction/normality with high nutrient levels (CN) through eating the high nutrient per calorie foods of the calorie normal **Plant Life Cycle Diet.**

By the way, the vegetarian California Seventh Day Adventists are as long lived or longer lived than the Okinawans who are known for longevity.

Many, in commenting on calorie restriction (actually CN), question if (so-called) restricted eating is worth the extra healthy years. Ask me on my early deathbed if I want to pig out on junk food one more time, or if I'd rather enjoy the company of my loved ones one more day.

Besides - with the calorie normal <u>Plant Life Cycle Diet</u> - **once you accustom your delicate little taste buds to a natural vegetable and fruit based diet there's no question of sensory deprivation**.

Threatened social deprivation maybe - but sensory deprivation no. Only the strong survive is true. **We simply have to be stronger in our resolve to live than to hang on to old eating and social-event habits**.

Sing A Song

To get you a little fired up about green leaves please sing the following to the tune of the philosophic song Row, Row, Row Your Boat:

Spinach, kale, cabbage, collard, boc choy, mustard, chard

> *Brussels sprouts, amaranth, Chinese cabbage, that wasn't very hard.*

Mazuna, sorrel, purslane, chicory, beat and turnip greens

> *Tat soi, sagen, pumpkin shoot greens by any means*

Tak choy, pac choy, watercress, dandelion you see

> *All these greens put here by God for eat by you and me.*   [Hawaiian version]

Then there's the lettuces - Romaine, etc, etc, sung to the tune of…

How about green leaf flavorings?   Basil, etc, etc. Chapter 8 is about spices, with a few recipe outlines. A full cookbook is available in late 2012.

We hardly realize how many green-leaf foods are available. All these green-leaf foods are so high in nutrients per calorie, it may be obvious they are meant to be a basis of the human (and primate) diet.

If you have a garden you know greens grow the fastest and are the first to be ready to eat by picking leaves or by harvesting the whole plant at once.

Per calorie density of nutrients is the key. Nutrients per calorie, not per gram, or per serving, or per portion - is the secret because the body reads calories, not grams. This is what the un-challenged calorie restriction (normality) studies reveal.

On first blush it seems that green leaves like Romaine lettuce aren't very dense. Well, they aren't very dense per pound. But as far as gaining or loosing weight goes our body reads calories.

Green leaves are incredibly nutrient dense per calorie, because the water in them that makes them, well... watery and not "dense", has no calories of course. They are also high volume, which fills your stomach.

In Chapter 8, The Flavors of India, the way is alluded to, to make green leaf and other plant parts in the **Plant Life Cycle Diet** taste great by spicing them in accordance with India's over five thousand year vegetarian tradition.

To find a shortcut to India to get their spices is the reason, after-all, Ye Olde Christopher Columbus (yea, I know he's an Italian who sailed for Spain) inadvertently discovered the "New World" for the Europeans. What else does the modern world owe to India? ... Someone said, "tech support".

Pytochemical research, and calorie restriction/ normality-inspired research are among the hottest areas of nutritional scientific study at the present time.

The pioneering calorie restriction / normality study of Clive McCay and colleagues M.F. Crowell and L.A. Maynard at Cornell University was published in 1935 in the *Journal of Nutrition.*

Recent research has shown that skipping meals, without restricting calories - in other words, "fast a while, eat a while", yields results similar to the now "traditional" CR/CN.

Increased irritability has been reported with alternate-day full-day fasts, but skipping a single meal is much less agitating.

"The [intermittently fed] mice are not calorie restricted, and yet we see changes in their physiology similar to those obtained with calorie restriction", neuroscientist Mark Mattson of the National Institute on Aging in Baltimore, Maryland told *Science News Online*.

Intermittent feeding also improved the animals' resistance to a neurotoxin that simulates Alzheimer's disease, the researchers report in the May 13, 2003 *Proceedings of the National Academy of Sciences*.

"When resting, rodents fed intermittently had lower heart rates and blood pressure and less circulating glucose and insulin in their blood than did the other rodents."

Which ever is best or if both together are best, it remains that when you eat you should choose foods according to their aggregate nutrients per calorie level, i.e. greens and buds, vegetable-fruits and sweet fruits first and foremost complimented by a few tubers & roots, legumes, and if desired whole grains.

The order of the plant life cycle.

Some of you may be familiar with the chart showing the comparison of nutrients between 100 calories of broccoli and 100 calories of steak.

Here it is:

	Broccoli	Steak
Calories	100	100
Protein (gm)	11 (2x)	5.4
Fiber (gm)	10.7	0
Vitamin A (IU)	6750 (281x)	24
Vitamin C (mg)	143	0
Vitamin E (IU)	26	0
Calcium (mg)	182 (75x)	2.4
Iron (mg)	2.2 (3X)	.7
Serving wt.	10 oz	.87 oz
Antioxi-Pytochem	very high	0

No comparison. Note serving weight of broccoli is 10 oz. To get equal protein from broccoli you only need half the serving weight of broccoli or 5 oz. Your stomach will be filled and hunger satisfied.

Because you will also be eating more calorie dense whole plant parts in addition to greens and broccoli buds, there is no problem of having to eat too much volume. Sweet potatoes for example, are more calorie-dense & have about 6.7% of calories from protein - slightly more than human mother's milk. How much protein is in human mother's milk?

What It Was

Look around outside. Chances are the numerically superior number of living elements you see are leaves. The same was true in distant, ancient times.

Wild, non-human animals, then as now, were relatively rarely seen. As a species, we grew up mostly eating high volume, high nutrient, low-calorie leaves and fruits.

If we descended from monkeys it makes sense – even though they, like us, are omnivores, they mostly eat leaves and fruits in the wild. If we have some other origin it still makes sense we ate leaves, as leaves are predominate in any original garden - whether Eden or Vrindavan.

Optional: http://en.wikipedia.org/wiki/Vrindavan.

Modern ideas of the superiority of high protein per gram foods, i.e. meat, fish, foul, eggs and dairy have been scientifically **disproved** in recent years. [See: The China Study, et al]

The idea of long, healthy, compassionate life through calorie restriction - actually calorie normality, is the main benefit of the calorie normal **Plant Life Cycle Diet**.

One can eat, say, half the calories of the Standard American Diet or the SAD, and get all the nutrients the body needs without the excess inflammatory "toxic" calories that cause premature cell aging, degenerative disease, and the unhealthy overweight condition. And without being hungry.

According to the **U.S. Department of Agriculture, Center for Nutrition Policy & Promotion** in 2005:

"It is important to focus on nutrient dense (ND) foods that deliver a high proportion of what your body needs for their amount of calories."

Here you see that the USDA knows the truth about the per **calorie** idea vs. the false per **gram** reporting that is done universally by almost all vested interests including they themselves the USDA.

Many people are concerned with getting enough protein. The essential amino acids that make up protein are not made by any animal or human body. They must be eaten or taken in by eating plant parts produced during the plant's life cycle. (or by eating a relatively few other non-animal living organisms, like nutritional yeast.)

All of the necessary essential amino acids are made by the action of sunlight on leaves. In the case of broccoli, as seen in the following chart, the leaves pass protein on to the broccoli buds.

The protein in steak or in any animal product is a processed food – processed by the animal's intestines. There's about 2x as much protein per calorie in romaine and in broccoli than in steak.

Both romaine and broccoli drive stakes into steak.

	Broccoli	Romaine	Steak
Calories	100	100	100
Protein (gm)	11	11.6 (2x)	5.4
Fiber (gm)	10.7	12	0
Cholesterol (mg)	0	0	55
Vitamin A (iu)	6750	18,570	24
Vitamin C (mg)	143	171	0
Vitamin E (IU)	26	3.2	0
Calcium (mg)	182	257	2.4
Antioxid - Phynutrs	very high	very high	0
Weight	10 oz	8 oz	1 oz

Note that leafy romaine has more protein and most other nutrients per calorie than broccoli. In all fairness T-bone steak does have a higher concentration of **one** of approximately **thirty** beneficial nutrients, per 100 calories, than broccoli, and that is Zinc with 1.44 mcg vs. 1.43 mcg for broccoli. All that .01 millionth of a gram difference in zinc is gained by only ingesting 2.93 gm per 100 calories of saturated fat in steak vs. .2 gm in broccoli - and 55 mg of cholesterol in steak vs. 0 mg in Broccoli.

(Calculated from www.foodgenius.com.)

Plus T-bone and other cuts of meat provide all those wonderful bovine antibiotics and growth hormones.

It is suspected that animal growth hormones may help cause premature puberty in human children, although that hasn't been proven yet scientifically - but hey, why take the risk?

Chicken and fish fare not much better. A little later I'll tell you about the latest story on fish and how fish eating is linked to breast cancer in women. I'm not jive'n you, or pushing some agenda - the science is there and most of the science is relatively recent.

A main problem in America today is that of overweight. You can see it - and the media are "Paul Revere-ing" the news.

The Eat Your Way To Health, Calorie Normal, Kind & Healthy, **Plant Life Cycle Diet** gives the scientifically substantiated nutrient-per-calorie IDEA it's public airing in a most palatable way especially in light of Chapter 8, "The Flavors of India." With the obesity epidemic in mind, anything that solves the national problem of excess calorie intake is welcome news.

Greens have about 100 calories per pound, so to eat the so-called average healthy diet of 2,000 calorie per day you would have to eat 20 pounds a day of greens - see you in the jungle. Wait - it's mostly water - see you at the urinal.

A healthful diet based on greens, vegetable-fruits and fruits, could not possibly make you fat if greens and fruits were the only things you ate. The calorie normal **Plant Life Cycle Diet** allows you to maintain calories at **normal** levels and increase nutrients without ever being hungry.

But since it is doubtful anyone could eat twenty pounds of greens a day, some less nutrient dense foods need to be eaten to decrease volume - and which also add flavor and variety; and balance out protein because greens are so high in protein - generally about 35 to 40% of calories.

Persons who maintain their healthy weight are fortunate indeed. They also prevent and reverse disease only by keeping their cholesterol below 150 total & 80 LDL with the **Plant Life Cycle Diet**.

Chapter 5

Fruits and Berries

Humans as a race have the ability to question what is the ultimate cause of and purpose for existence. The humble position is that somewhere there are persons who somehow know the answer. At least we know we can inquire.

By many measures of common sense we might say fruit is the most obvious food for humans. By sight, by taste & by smell, by modern research and by ancient wisdom fruit is food for humans.

You always see young children's play toys as bright yellows, reds, oranges and blues - just like the colors of bananas, apples, oranges and grapes - **the colors of the rainbow**!

It may not be an accident that a banana turns yellow when ripe, and then even begins to get cute little black dots on it when at its peak of ripeness.

Do tomatoes turn red by accident when they are ripe and ready to be eaten? Oranges turn green to orange? Strawberries? Mangos? On and on. Color change in fruits when they ripen alerts color vision-ed humans when to harvest and eat - what a nice touch.

According to the first study done in this area by Tufts University, the fruits with the highest nutrients per calorie including phyto-chemicals were blueberries, blackberries, raspberries and strawberries. All darkly colored berries. The same is generally true in greens - the darker the color, the more nutrients per calorie. Newer studies that include more fruits have a few other fruits rated slightly higher than blueberries.

As always, one must be aware of **the difference between nutrients per gram and per calorie** – per calorie being the accurate one. Most studies are still done per gram and are misleading and have to be manually recalculated to per-calorie, to give the true picture.

The latest science tells us that the phyto-pigments found especially in the skins of fruits protect us from cancer. Fruits have about two to three times the calories per pound as greens. Because of their powerful cancer protective properties fruits are heartily recommended in plentiful amounts in the Taste The Rainbow **Plant Life Cycle Diet** – wouldn't be the rainbow without 'em.

Chapter 6
Tubers & Legumes Yes, Grains & Nuts Maybe

Next in ranking in the fountain of youth, calorie normal, Taste The Rainbow, **Plant Life Cycle Diet** are tubers & roots, then beans and lastly grains.

As reported by ABC News some time ago (2000), in the village of Yuzuri Hara, Japan, people routinely live to the age of **100 with soft, un-aged, smooth looking skin.** Their secret?

In place of eating grains they eat guess what? Tubers and roots. Cooked but unprocessed tuber and root crops. Again most "roots" we eat are botanically underground swollen stem-tubers and root-tubers.

Unlike other regions of Japan that grow rice, Yuzuri Hara's hilly terrain is better suited to growing and harvesting root crops, including different sweet potatoes, corms like taro and dasheen & various sticky white potatoes some of which, that when cooked taste similar to regular old Idaho potatoes.

Because of hyaluronic acid in sweet potatoes and potatoes, it's probable that the beautiful skin of each of the residents of Yuzuri Hara is prevented from aging by eating these root crops in the place of eating grains.

Prepared grains taste good but are only borderline nutrient dense having relatively high calories, and they have anti-nutrients. Maybe that's part of the reason why you always hear the phrase, "Stop eating bread!"

The temporary weight loss success of the Atkins Diet and similar low-carbohydrate diets is due to restricting lots of fractionated white flower and sugary processed foods.

In the Japanese version of the calorie normal **Plant Life Cycle Diet,** certain root crops like sweet potatoes (satsumaimo), sticky white potatoes (satoimo); and other potato roots and tubers (including imoji), are rated high in nutrient value, and have skin, joint and other anti-aging properties especially when grains are omitted from one's diet.

Sweet potatoes in general have good nutrient per calorie ratios, slightly better than grains, but are not acid forming like grains.

Again, many of the so-called roots we eat – like potatoes and sweet potatoes - are specialized underground food storage **stem-tubers** or **root-tubers**; or like the onion - are balls of specialized underground **leaves**.

But always remember that greens, vegetable-fruits and sweet fruits are our staples. Greens are the towering giants of what we should eat for maximum health, longevity, weight loss & beauty - for maximum everything. Closely followed by vegetable-fruits like green beans, snap peas, zucchini, cucumbers etc; and sweet fruits – followed by more calorie-dense sweet potatoes and legumes. More on legumes soon.

If gaining weight is your problem, greens are your friend, and grains, especially processed ones with added oil, sugar and/or salt, are your enemy. Grains also have anti-nutrients like **lectins, gluten, and phytate**.

Eat More Fruits & Vegetables Is Wrong Advice

Remember we said the phrase: "Eat more fruits and vegetables" is inaccurate?

Well first of all it should be: "Eat more green vegetables, bud-vegetables, vegetable-fruits and sweet fruits".

But also it means, or should mean: DO NOT EAT - meat, fish, foul, eggs, oil, and dairy.

As noted previously if we add more of anything to what we're eating now, we'll just keep getting fatter.

No, no, no. We certainly don't want that, now do we?

Of course not.

"Eat More Fruits and Vegetables" is basically food industry allowed half-truth B.S. and we don't want to step in that.

Eat Less Vs. Addiction

The problem with the statement - "Eat Less" in reference to heavy foods - is that because **food is addictive according to the calories per bite** so to speak, it's virtually impossible to "eat less." It would be better to not use **any, zero -** just like tobacco, or napalm bombs for example.

In the vast, vast, vast majority of cases no one can STOP being addicted to drinking or smoking unless they teetotal (stop completely).

Teetotal one day at a time for enough days in a row and the cravings will go away (between instantly, and twelve weeks time).

Thinking: "Oh, I'll have a little of this, or a little of that once in a while", soon leads to falling off the wagon.

Moderation and Balanced Diet B.S.

The phrases: "All things in moderation" and "Balanced diet" similarly, are misleading in the case of healthy diet.

As to "Moderation": In ancient times when food was generally scarce, we could eat <u>high</u> calorie, low nutrient foods when they were available and not get addicted because the next day they weren't available.

In modern developed countries rich, heavy foods are being pushed and are available everywhere **precisely because they are addictive and have longer shelf lives, and because manufacturers and marketers profit from you being addicted.**

Buyer beware.

Just for fun - where exactly is the balance point in a healthy balanced diet? Look at the clipped **Plant Life Cycle Diet** chart below:

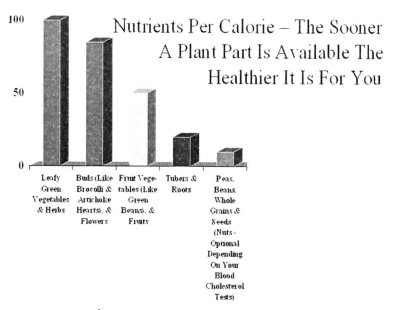

About here ⇑.

Balanced diet should **not** mean: "Eat a little bit of everything good and bad." In our opulent environment, the high calorie, low nutrient foods deleted from the **right side** of the chart have us physically addicted to, and eating off of that side of the chart.

The opposite of what is naturally good for us.

Again - in ancient times food was scarce and that was the problem. Today junk foods, high fat plant foods, and rich unhealthy animal foods are super-abundant and available. Addiction fueled by super-abundance is the problem. **Addiction is a strong force.** The solution is to eat **zero** animal products and junk.

The easiest way to improve your diet is to t-total all of the full chart's right-side animal and junk "foods" all at once or at least one category at a time, step-by-step starting from the far right side of the chart. (Full chart on page 47.)

In today's environment that IS the only way!

The Only Way To Eat Only Vegetables & Fruits - Is To <u>BUY</u> Only Vegetables & Fruits

And to not eat any – zero of the other unhealthy things.

The ignorant and/or deceitful are epidemic, and will directly and indirectly try to dissuade you from the healthiest eating.

You may feel like you're being persecuted, ridiculed and cast out... Don't worry - you *are* being persecuted, ridiculed and cast out.

But with support and association - by personal contact, electronically or by other means - with other like-minded persons, you can and will succeed. Email me at: mdasNow@gmail.com.

As Gloria Sorensen of the **Dana-Farber Cancer Institute** said: "Family members, friends and coworkers have the potential to play an important role in determining the climate of health behaviors, such as eating habits."

Tell your friends about this book, tell your family about whole, high nutrient greens, buds, vegetable-fruits and fruits, and eat zero processed and animal foods - and get their support and cooperation.

At least get their willingness to tolerate your healthy desire and not be anti-parties. Most importantly find an enthusiastic diet and lifestyle **buddy** or two.

My wife Sunanda Dasi and I have developed various weekend retreats and multi-day "boot camps" where students can come for intense training and to make new like-minded friends.

If you are interested, send us an email at: mdasNow@gmail.com for future event dates, or for personal counseling, support, shepherding and/or guidance.

How To Do It

It's simple to succeed… but challenging. The steps are easy to hear but harder to do. But you can do it.

First is knowledge. Second is determination. Third and in the long run perhaps most important is support.

One-cup knowledge, two-cups determination and three-cups support.

Modern & Ancient Eaters Of Soothing Alkaline Tubers & Roots

Getting back to the topic at hand, this chapter is about roots, and tubers like sweet potatoes, and about legumes.

To review a bit - tubers and roots are soothing alkaline instead of inflammatory acid forming – that's good for you. (pages 17-18)

Villagers in Yuzuri Hara, Japan live to 100 with **smooth unwrinkled skin** by eating various sweet potatoes in place of grains – that's very good.

Now, beginning about 1980 scientists at Harvard, Yale, Penn State and from other institutions determined that Australopithecus, the first human ancestor to walk upright, probably added roots and tubers to the chimp, gorilla and monkey diet of mostly green vegetables and fruits.

Not only Australopithecus, but also it was proposed that tubers and roots (scientifically called **USO**'s for underground storage organs) are responsible for the rise of **modern** man.

Don't believe it? Here's an online address of the full 2002 study from scientists at the University of Minnesota and Harvard University titled: **"The rise of the hominids as an adaptive shift in fallback foods: Plant underground storage organs (USOs) and Australopith origins."**

[If the link is dead google the title.] http://gregladen.com/wordpress/wp-content/pdf/Laden_Wrangham_Roots.pdf

Now, I'm the first one to doubt what someone says happened a million years ago (I can't remember what happened yesterday) so I would rely somewhat more on the recent Yuzuri Hara revelation and other recent science.

The upshot of all this, in light of Yuzuri Hara, in light of calorie restriction/normality, and in light of the anti-nutrients in grains - is to chose tubers over grains when you have a choice - for health, beauty, smooth unwrinkled skin, and long life.

Legumes

The following chart from 2008 shows that a plant-based diet that included legumes was common to the diet of all **three** of the longest-lived populations.

Grains were common to only **two** of the three, and nuts were a significant part of only **one** of the populations.

This is in line with what has been reported in this book – namely that grains are less desirable than legumes, and that nuts are less desirable than grains. The order of desirability of these three types of seeds - from more desirable to less desirable is: legumes, grains, nuts. This is the hierarchy of seeds.

(The hierarchy of desirability of starches highest to lowest is: tubers, legumes, grains.)

In view of the above, and with reference to calorie restriction/calorie normality, and with reference to the fact that a total blood cholesterol level below 150 mg/dL, in combination with an LDL level below 80, makes you degenerative-disease-proof - it has been recommended in this book to base your consumption of nuts (assuming compliance with all the other recommendations herein) upon **your own particular blood test results**.

Here is the long life populations chart: (Loma Linda residents are 7th Day Adventists.)

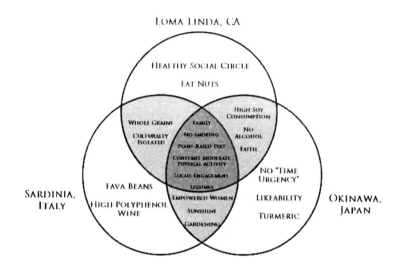

Although these were among the longest-lived peoples, with the addition and observance of the modern scientific information detailed in this book these people - **and you** - can live even longer happy, healthy, cognizant and compassionate lives.

A note here is although legumes are acid forming and calcium leaching in the body - they are apparently healthy when grains are minimized and net acid balance pressures are kept low.

In addition to leaching calcium from your bones, eating too much acid forming food also causes muscle wasting as we age. So be careful, and you may want to be sure to eat alkaline sweet potatoes.

Chapter 7

Mr. B12, Sir Omega-3 & Dr. D

Deserving of special mention is Vitamin B12 an essential vitamin that doesn't originate from plants or animals but from bacteria.

Due to modern sanitary living this vitamin is lacking in many diets. Vitamin B12 pill supplements are the best source of B12 – 1000 mcg once a week to start and then 2000 mcg once a month after you blood levels are solidly in the center of the reference range. Among many other critically important things, B-12 reportedly also helps keep your hair from turning gray.

B12 containing Red Star Vegetarian Support Nutritional Yeast and other nutritional yeasts available in most health food stores, and possibly in regular supermarkets, are secondary sources of Vitamin B12 (and tastes like cheese).

Omega-3, an essential fat we don't get a high enough proportion of (in relationship to Omega-6) in the modern diet, is found in abundance in flax seed meal & purslane.

"Jonny's Selected Seeds" has various purslane seeds at:
http://www.johnnyseeds.com/search.aspx?SearchTerm=purslane .

Purslane is one of the best foods you never ate. They can be continuously harvested during the growing season. The wild variety, I think tastes a little better.

Ground flaxseed also contains breast and colon cancer tumor shrinking (reported) lignan in high quantities. A maximum of two level teaspoons a day.

Because I don't eat any oil (or nuts, most of which have high amounts of omega-6, and significant amounts of yes - saturated fat in them) – and I do eat lots of greens, which have ideal omega-3 to omega-6 ratios in them, I personally no longer take flaxseed meal regularly– just eat greens and grow my own purslane which is super easy to grow.

Flax **oil** is not recommended for various reasons, except temporarily in special rare circumstances - mainly because oil is a processed food and damages the blood vessels. More on oil damage later.

Blood levels of long chain DHA omega-3 fat have recently been shown to be highest in Vegans, higher than meat-eaters and much higher than vegetarians – how about that!

See:
http://www.ajcn.org/content/92/5/1040.short

Taking fish oil to get DHA omega-3, is like smoking cigarettes to get the vitamins that are in tobacco.

Even in the vested drug, supplement and surgery industry, the fish oil myth is now beginning to be slowly chipped away. A study published April 9, 2012 in the Archives of Internal Medicine states that there is "no conclusive evidence" for recommending fish oil to prevent a first or subsequent heart attack.

As might be expected vested influences minimize and challenge the findings. Snake oil salesmen, educators and suppliers die hard.

As for Dr. D - vitamin D – for most people just get sufficient sunshine **without burning!** If you live in northern latitudes and don't get out in the summer you might want to take a vitamin D supplement. Or move to Hawaii.

Have your vitamin-D blood level checked if you don't get out in the sun regularly.

Chapter 8

The Flavors of India

We can be addicted in the world, first and foremost to the desire for sense gratification. All these greens and fruits in the **Plant-Life Cycle Diet** that could appear to the uninformed, to be a little monotonous consumed in staple amounts - may need to be spiced up a little bit.

Good fortune has it that there exists naturally many good tasting green leaf and other high taste spices to help.

There are many high-taste-per-calorie items in all categories of foods in the **Plant Life Cycle Diet** to aid in flavoring and spicing.

Variety is the spice of life. And spice definitely helps in producing a great variety of desirable tastes in the **Plant Life Cycle Diet**.

Did you ever see the movie: "The Little Princess"? In that movie there is a beautiful scene where the two little girl stars of the film are in India situated upon the head of a great statue, which is partially submerged in a beautiful tropical water pond. The camera sweeps around the two little girls as sunlight streams through the jungle foliage.

India is at once the land of God, demi-gods and spices.

The oldest continuous developed culture on this little Planet Earth, India is the original vegetarian culture, complete with a dramatic spiritual heritage contained in voluminous Scripture.

Columbus was looking for a shortcut to India and its spices for the sense gratification of European royalty. Unique and tasteful spice flavorings are quite the thing even among us peasants.

You can live like a "Royal" by eating the **Plant Life Cycle Diet** and by learning the spicing and flavoring techniques hinted at in the following recipes outlines:

Royal Romaine Salad

Finely chopped romaine lettuce, tomato, cucumber & onion, sprinkled with Red Star vegetarian support nutritional yeast, a few drops of lemon juice, a bit of mustard sauce, a pinch of asafetida and if desired a tiny pinch of iodized salt or Dulse flakes. (Taking no salt in canned and packaged foods allows for a tiny pinch of salt in home cooking or added at the table.)

Bypass Proof Broccoli

Quick-cooked in a little water cut broccoli, cumin, ginger, a few chopped onions and a tiny pinch of iodized salt.

Spinach With Spiced Green Beans

Half blended, half not blended spinach (lightly cooked or not cooked), and chopped crunchy long green beans with mustard, black pepper, asafetida, cumin and if desired a tiny pinch of salt.

Peas, Potatoes And Cauliflower

Cooked peas, cauliflower, cubed potato and/or purple sweet potato, with turmeric, garam masala and dill weed.

Mashed Brussels Sprouts With Cut Mung Bean Sprouts

Cooked mashed Brussels Sprouts, cut bean sprouts, with **no-oil** home made pasta sauce with Italian spice.

Mixed Fruit Two Banana Smoothie With Cardamom Or Rose Water

Strawberry, papaya, two banana smoothie blended in the smallest possible amount of water with cinnamon, cardamom and/or rose water.

Green Beans With Pasta Sauce & Sweet Potatoes or Potatoes

Boiled chopped green beans and sweet potatoes or potatoes with non-GMO, no-oil home made pasta sauce.

Notice that a dark leafy, or solid green vegetable or fruit is the main ingredient in all of the above preparations.

Cook Book

The art and science of preparing and spicing plant–based, **Plant Life Cycle Diet Cuisine** is extensive and will be beautifully detailed in the as previously mentioned full cookbook.

If you would like to be added to the availability notification list, please send an email with the words "Cook Book" in the subject line to: mdasNow@gmail.com.

Chapter 9

And In the End

If you don't buy it or accept it as a gift you can't eat it. So in a way, this is where the main battle is fought. Just keep chanting, "Something green, something green, give me something green – and some fruit."

Make your shopping list with the words -- Green leaf, bud-vegetables, vegetable-fruits and fruit – first & foremost, at the top, in large letters. Then below that -- flavorings and spices. If you pick up a bag of chips, catch yourself and put them back down, muttering: "Green! Green!! Green!!!"

When you prepare foods think green leaf, buds, vegetable-fruits, and fruits as main dishes – tubers & roots, and legumes as side dishes. And whole grains in small amounts daily - and generously on bona fide holidays, weddings and feast days.

"Side dishes" means small portions about one-third the size or less of the green and other vegetables on your plate.

A more detailed breakdown of proportions is coming up.

For now you could have, say, two main green dishes - one maybe a salad, the other maybe lightly boiled and spiced broccoli or a leafy vegetable sprinkled with Red Star brand Vegetarian Support Formula nutritional yeast added at the table to avoid heating which destroys vitamin B12; plus a side of sweet potatoes maybe blended into a poi, with a little bit of fruit as desert each day.

You may like to make more of the green and vegetable-fruit dishes than you can eat so that you always have green dish and vegetable dish leftovers EASILY AVAILABLE the next day.

When someone offers you junk food or low nutrient chump change animal food – some refusal lines could be: "Thanks but I just ate a big meal." Or: "Thanks so much but I'm watching my diet." Or even: "Thanks but I'm allergic to Twinkies", or what ever it is.

Another important consideration for many people is **ease and quickness of preparation**. Most preparations in the **Plant Life Cycle Diet** are quick and easy to prepare using fresh or frozen vegetables.

An Indian style stainless steal spice container is a great time saver that encourages spice use and creative experimentation. Call my wife Sunanda at 808-878-6821 and ask about this.

A slightly controversial but very easy way to prepare foods in the **Plant Life Cycle Diet** is to use **no salt added** canned vegetables.

Two somewhat recent studies, one by the University of Illinois and one by the University of Massachusetts, reported that the nutrients per calorie of canned foods were in most cases equal to or occasionally more than fresh or frozen vegetables. <u>The studies were funded by the canning industry so they may or may not be biased</u>.

It was stated that this is possible because **canning stops vitamin loss** at the time of canning which is very soon after harvesting, whereas commercially produced "fresh" vegetables spend more time from harvest through shipping to your table.

... And because the vegetables, fruits and beans grown for canning can be of a different, **better type and picked closer to ripening** than the "fresh" produce grown to withstand long transport and to have long shelf-life times.

Eating a commercially produced, non-organic, canned, no added salt vegetable is better than eating <u>any</u> chump change animal or fractionated/processed food.

By the way, slaughterhouse products like blood, bones, brains and feathers are used in **commercial organic** & **home organic** fertilizer.

Royal Problem

As stated in the book, *The Pleasure Trap* by Doctors Lisle & Goldhamer, the United States has no hereditary royalty, but in the 20th century via film, radio and television a new royalty was born. One particular person became the first king of rock & roll.

This particular person by his kingship, gained access to pleasures once only available to hereditary kings and queens.

Unfortunately, he succumbed to the disease of kings: over-indulgence. Who is or was that king?

Elvis Presley's life is a metaphor to modern western civilization that in the mid and latter part of the 20th century - through amazing advancement of technology - began to produce a super-abundance of low cost, easily available calorie-heavy foods; and lots of drugs.

In the modern world we're surrounded by - and bombarded with advertisements for these calorie-heavy unhealthy foods - and at the same time we are told to "eat right". But do we really know how to eat right? No we don't… and here's why. (Well you do now if you've been listening.)

We are being tricked by vested interests into NOT knowing clearly - exactly what are healthy foods, and what are **un**healthy foods.

We are being confused by vested interests into not knowing what is the easy-to-understand, simple and clear, proper order of desirability of foods, i.e. exactly what is bad, what is good, what is better and what is best.

And we are being fooled by vested interests into denying the simple and only permanent solution to the problem of our actual physical addiction to easy-to-consume unhealthy calorie-heavy foods - **zero.**

What's the common four letter word that begins with a J – and ends with -unk for easy-to-consume unhealthy calorie-heavy foods?

As an historical survival mechanism we are easily addicted to rich foods by evolution - but technology, supermarkets & fast-food drive-throughs have changed things - so that our survival instinct to prefer high calorie foods, is no longer healthy for us. Please allow me to repeat:

Our problem is that we are physically **addicted** to super-available heart attack, cancer, stroke, diabetes, Alzheimer's and many other disease-causing calorie-heavy animal and processed foods, promoted and actually glorified - or ignored, as the case may be - by some powerful and sometimes not-so-benign vested interests. We are in denial.

Here's the **Total Problem** stated in the simplest terms:

#1) We are absolutely physically addicted to unhealthy foods – **that's why we're still eating them thinking life would loose some pleasure if you couldn't have them once in a while**. They give a rush like addictive drugs do.

It's a full-on physical addiction, neurologically exactly like cigarettes or any other addictive drug.

#2) All-pervading powerful vested interests in society - many that are supposed to be protecting you, don't actually - consciously or unconsciously - want you to stop eating unhealthy foods.

According to the **International Journal of Obesity** December 2007 issue - Susan Roberts, PhD director of the USDA Energy Metabolism Laboratory stated:

"The most identifiable thing about the foods people **crave** is that they are highly dense in calories".

Crave means addicted. They know it's an addiction – it's not a free choice. It is known.

Later you'll learn **how to overcome** our biggest problem - **the addiction problem**.

The problem government and industry knows about - but won't tell you straight. That's later.

Much information about the complicity of vested interests is revealed in the 2004 Peter Jennings / ABC News documentary on the USDA's food subsidy program and how it **promotes** disease - and on advertising of unhealthy foods to children.

Below are web addresses 1 & 2 for **short** audio clips to listen to now of that documentary:

In the first clip 1, Peter is talking about the two images you see below.

1. http://www.MadhavaDas.com/pj1.mp3

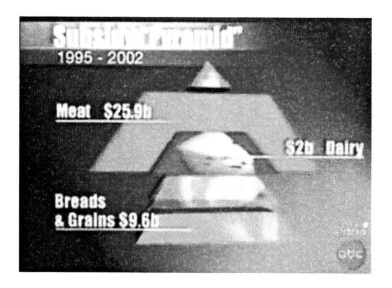

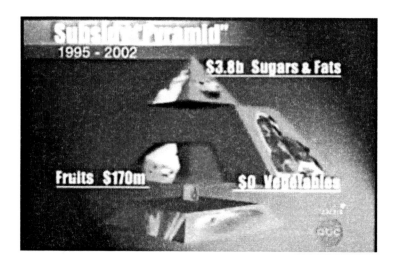

In the next **short** clip 2, you'll hear about complicity by food manufacturers & the <u>advertising</u> industry.

2. <u>http://www.MadhavaDas.com/pj2.mp3</u>

That's the processed food & advertising industries and the government that consciously don't want you to stop eating unhealthy foods.

Down below is a link to the full 42-minute audio of the program titled "How the food industry is deceiving you". You are requested to listen to it at your convenience.

Like most "health" websites, there is a small amount of good nutritional info at the below site, but mostly a lot of ultimately confusing half-truth. Stick with me, and ask me anything to clarify any question you have.

Contact me at <u>mdasNow@gmail.com</u>.

<u>http://transitionnow.wordpress.com/2011/04/0 8/video-how-the-food-industry-is-deceiving- you-with-peter-jennings/</u> If the link is dead, google the title: How the food industry is deceiving you.

Who are some other complicit vested interests?

How about the pharmaceutical industry – "Side effects include vomiting, diarrhea & death."

How about the medical industry – hospitals & doctors make their living from your sickness.

The federal government is a very large landowner & there are also very many large powerful private landowners – for ease of operation, they love to just graze cattle on their land.

Then there are well-funded food company and many other industry lobbyists in Washington DC.

Can you think of any more vested interests? … I just thought of one: HMO's - the medical insurance industry - if you weren't sick all the time - they'd have less business too.

So many vested interests profit from your sickness.

Here's a quiz question for you: What innocent people do junk food manufacturers like to advertise to?

By the way, you're cordially invited to send in your heartfelt testimonials & comments about this book by email to: mdasNow@gmail.com. Include your photo and you'll receive a free subscription to the monthly Plant Life Cycle Diet email newsletter.

Plant Life Cycle Diet

In 1935 Dr. Clive McCay of Cornell University did the first calorie restriction study on rodents that variously increased vigorous healthy lifespan up to 60%. Here's a link to Dr McCay's Wikipedia page:

http://en.wikipedia.org/wiki/Clive_McCay

As previously mentioned, the National Institute on Aging, National Institutes Of Health in 2007 said:

"Dietary caloric restriction (CR) is the **only** intervention repeatedly demonstrated to retard the onset and incidence of age-related diseases, maintain function, and extend both lifespan and health span in mammals, including brain and behavioral function."

If you haven't looked already, here again at: http://www.MadhavaDas.com/primate.gif you can see the above quote as part of the National Institute on Aging's report on the primates study of calorie restriction.

The up to 60% increase in vibrant lifespan we're talking about is not possible by merely exercising (although **along with** the Plant Life Cycle Diet exercising helps), not by taking vitamins & not by taking supplements.

Have you ever heard of resveritrol? For those who haven't: Resveritrol has recently in a very limited way, been shown to extend healthy lifespan in one insect and in one worm species, but **not** in mice. A further limitation is that the study on resveritrol was done using extremely high dosages.

What high dosage resveritrol does to HUMANS has never been determined and is totally unknown. So don't believe MARKETER'S claims just yet about resveritrol. More on this later.

A normal mouse lives about 28 months. See chart below.

Total Average Life Span of CR Mice vs. Non-CR Mice

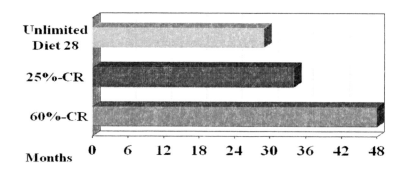

At 60% restriction a mouse's average lifespan is about 48 months.

One thing to note here is that the percent of vibrant life-span extension is about equal to the percent of calorie restriction.

But the most important thing about CR – the thing that vested interests usually ignore completely - is that **nutrient** levels are maintained at **normal** levels. So Calorie Restriction could also be called Nutrient Normality. More on this later.

If anyone would like to see a picture of the world's oldest living mouse you can see'em at:

www.MadhavaDas.com/oldestmouse.htm - go there now!

Below you see a chart showing human life expectancy extension, extrapolated from mice to men.

Extrapolation From Mice to Men
Human Life Span

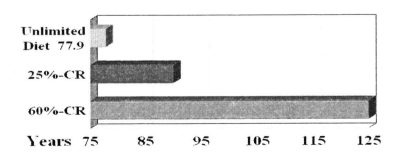

Washington University School Of Medicine in 2004 said of 18 persons following a CR diet for from 2 to 10 years: "The participant's blood pressure averaged that of a healthy 10 year old even though the subjects ranged in age from 35 to 82."

In the Honolulu Heart Program Study in 2004 Dr. Bradley Wilcox said of 1915 men whose calorie intake was observed over a 36 year period: "This first large human study confirms theories suggested in 1935 by the first animal studies."

National Academy Of Sciences 2001 Dr. Stephen Spindler said: "Mice on only one month of a very low-calorie [and high nutrient] diet reversed close to 70% of the genome changes induced by age."

It's never too late to start.

Calorie Normality

Want to know what vested interests are doing with this knowledge? They're calling calorie restriction a "starvation diet".

If this were starvation, how can all living beings tested, live a vibrant 50% longer? That's not starvation. That's prosperity.

The point is, no one is starving – the fact is - that everyone is very healthy and happy. Remember that nutrients are not restricted. You'll learn more about this in a little bit.

In long-time historical terms, what today's devious vested interest status quo calls "restriction" or "starvation" - is actually our quite comfortable NORMALITY - since time immemorial!

Let's restate that because it's critical: What today's vested interests are trying to scare you with by calling it starvation or restriction, is **not** starvation or restriction - but is the **totally normal pattern** humans have been quite happy and prosperous with for thousands and thousands of years.

Calorie Restriction is actually Calorie Normality and Nutrient Normality - and after withdrawing from addiction to artificially calorie dense foods - Calorie Normality feels quite... well... NORMAL! And Happy!

Essential Amino Acids Come From Plants

Another big point... All essential amino acids needed to make up all types of protein are created - in the leaves of plants – that's where they appear on this planet, that's where they originate – that's where they come from.

The protein in meat and fish flesh is first processed through the animal's stomach and intestines, and tends to have harmful sulfur compounds.

Essential amino acids have their pure origin in the leaves of plants.

It is a myth that plant protein is incomplete protein. Plant protein is complete protein and is actually the highest quality protein.

Vested interests, including food companies, advertising companies, drug companies and all their lobbyists, that are almost unimaginably powerful and devious lately, take minor scientific points and very deftly twist and distort things to bamboozle you into believing that animal protein is necessary and is healthier than plant protein.

If you want to read much more about animal protein please read the Cornell University, Oxford University, China Study reported in the 400 page best selling book simply called: *The China Study*.

Essential Amino Acids Originate In Leaves

Leaves average about 35-40% protein by calorie measurement. And if there's one thing, those in the know, know - it's that Calorie Restriction errr Calorie Normality studies have revealed that NUTRIENTS SHOULD BE MEASURED PER CALORIE - <u>NOT</u> PER GRAM OR PER SERVING (i.e. per bite) - AS IS ALMOST UNIVERSALLY DONE BY VESTED INTERESTS.

The fact that nutrients should be measured per calorie, not per gram is a big **un**reported revelation of Calorie Restriction studies.

Excess calories are toxic. All nutrients should be measured per calorie by truthful interests, not against gram weight or "serving size" as vested interests do.

Gram weight measurements – as you'll see very shortly in some charts - and serving size measurements **distort the understanding of what are healthy and what are unhealthy**

foods – much to the delight of those who want to kill you for their own economic gain.

Strong words?   Heart attacks, cancer, strokes, diabetes and Alzheimer's disease are strong diseases.

Another bamboozle vested interests throw at you to disparage so-called Calorie Restriction, really Calorie Normality – is that they say it may work by putting stress on your body.   If you've ever over-eaten you know that's what puts stress on your body. Over-eating. Not normal eating.

Un-addicted normal eating - what they cheatingly call starvation – takes stress off your body.   Un-addicted, normal eating, which almost no one in the modern world does any more, takes all the stress off your body.

Nutrient levels compared to calories - is what is critically important. And not to eat heavy foods.

It turns out that most all nutrients appear & are created in leaves of plants. Green leafy vegetables are HIGHEST in nutrients & LOWEST in calories.

Green leafy vegetables have the highest nutrient to calorie ratio. Green leafy vegetables have the highest nutrient density & are the healthiest foods - by far. **Green** leafy vegetables & some solid bud-vegetables including things like broccoli, and the **RAINBOW of vegetable-fruits and fruits** are our STAPLE foods.

Looking at the **Nutrient Density Per Calorie** chart below, nutrient density per calorie occurs on a continuum or hierarchy going downward from the leaf according to the plant's reproductive life cycle.

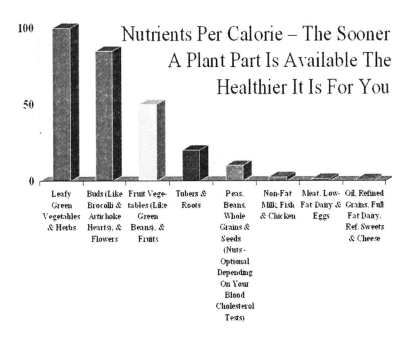

In other words - leafy and solid bud-vegetables have the highest nutrient density per calorie - by far - followed by vegetable-fruits and sweet fruits.

The vested interests' food group, pyramid and new food plate ideas do not present the truth revealed in the Nutrient Density Per Calorie Continuum or Hierarchy chart.

Repeating what was said earlier in the book - the idea of food groups is like the idea that the earth is flat. "Food groups" is a false idea and is outdated, dangerous and misleading - and the vested interests use the outdated idea of food groups to mislead, confuse and bamboozle you.

Again, this is deliberate on their part and very irresponsible - as are the quotes "find the right balance" and "all things in moderation". **If it's bad - zero is the right amount.**

I apologize for all this repetition & negativity but really as I'm remembering this again here - I'm **feeling** the irresponsibility of the vested interests. And it's making me sad and a little angry.

Here are B-9 folate and calcium charts comparing per gram vs. per calorie. B-9 Folate is necessary for the production and maintenance of new cells and also needed for DNA replication.

B-9 Folate Comparison

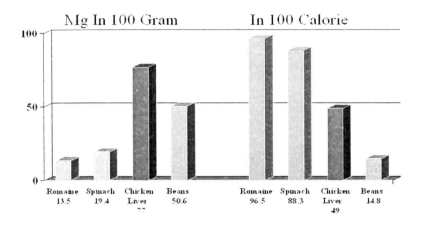

Honest per calorie determination turns bogus per gram calculations on their head.

Calcium Comparison

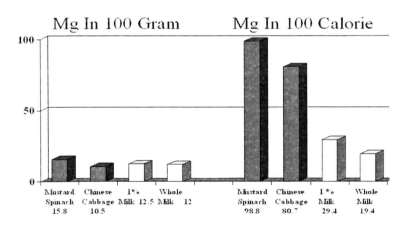

Per gram, calcium is about the same — but look what happens when we see it per calorie on the right side of the above chart.

Per gram, fish has the same amount of cholesterol as meat.

But in the per calorie comparison - look at this:

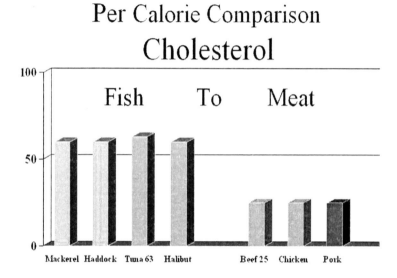

Fish is not healthy – not even in "moderation".

Here's a "fish are not vegetables" Dilbert cartoon:

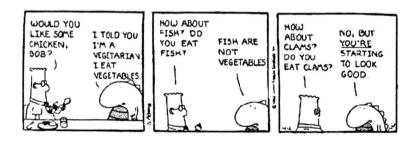

More on fish later.

Shaky Pyramids & Cracked Plates

Now you're going to hear about shaky pyramids, cracked plates and other false concepts.

Remember the quote from the **U.S. Department of Agriculture Center for Nutrition Policy & Promotion 2005:**

"It is important to focus on nutrient dense (ND) foods that deliver a high proportion of what your body needs for their amount of calories."

Again - the USDA knows the truth about the per calorie idea vs. the mistaken and false per gram reporting that is done universally by almost all vested interests including they themselves - the USDA.

The Nutrient Density Per Calorie **Continuum** seen in the following first chart reflects the **Plant Life Cycle Diet** and represents truth.

The somewhat recent USDA food-group-based food pyramids and now plates - seen successively further below - represent falsehood and partial-truth.

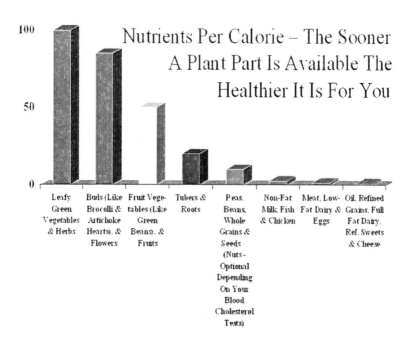

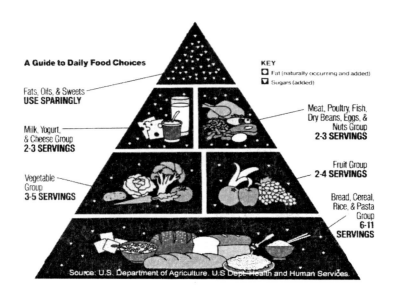

The 1992 above, and somewhat recent government food pyramid below, depict bogus food groups - circumventing the nutrient density per calorie **continuum hierarchy** at the expense of your health.

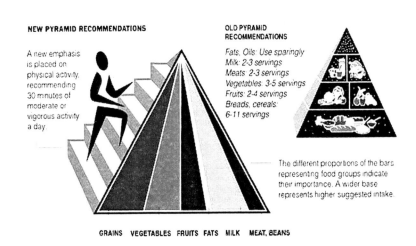

Government and industry half-truths are more dangerous than outright falsehoods because they are more devious and misleading.

In their vertical lie... whoops - pyramid, they sneakily made milk bigger than vegetables and almost equal to grains.

Vested interests build shaky pyramids.

That was the old sound byte for this book.

And as of June 2011, the USDA is trying to keep cracked plates spinning on shaky sticks.

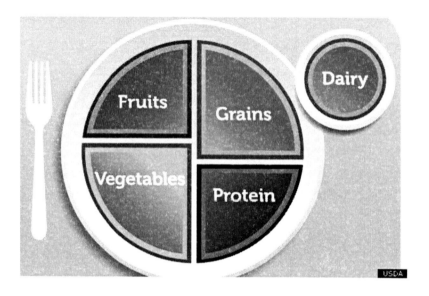

A much more pleasing depiction - but still not accurate enough.

The inclusion of dairy is one of the two big problems of the plate depiction. The other is more subtle in the form of the word "Protein". As the word protein is synonymous with "meat" in the popular mind, the plate depiction allows for and does nothing to warn against eating meat.

The new sound byte is: Cracked plates don't hold water.

Exploiting Pinocchio

Listen for yourself as you play a now slightly outdated but still illuminating relatively recent radio spot from some corrupted offending vested interests:

http://www.MadhavaDas.com/pino.mp3

Really, please do this now.

I started to cry when I heard this advertisement on the radio when I realized what was happening.

"The right balance of everything you and your child need" and what follows that, is false and misleading.

They have even corrupted Pinocchio – it's almost beyond belief.

They have actually taken a beloved cartoon character famous for learning to tell the truth, and used him to pervert truth for economic gain, and to maintain their favored position in the vested status quo - all at your expense and at the children's expense.

Despicable indeed.

The Truth: Eat Your Way To Health Plant Life Cycle Diet

You now know the truth about how vested interests have conspired to mislead and confuse you in the past. Rest assured they will continue trying in the future.

And you also now know, the most advanced, complete and honest understanding of healthy eating - the **Plant Life Cycle Diet.**

With your new knowledge of vested interests, you may now have some doubts about wine study, and supplement advertiser's Resveritrol claims of longevity simply by taking a pill without any rules, boundaries and limitations on eating disease causing unhealthy foods, that all those vested interests want you to keep eating. Or by removing certain aged cells from prematurely aged mice. Nothing else except calorie restriction is proven now, or in view of the time it would take, could be proven in humans for a long time from now.

Knowing the truth - there remains one big personal problem. In just one moment you'll learn more truth about how to overcome our one big personal health problem - THE BIG PROBLEM of **addiction** to the junk-food pusher's fare.

Cooking Courses

In the future, my wife Sunanda and I - Sunanda is from India, I'm from Pennsylvania - my wife and I may be offering live telephone, or live online video Eat Your Way To Health cooking courses; and live telephone, or live online video Healthy Indian 100% Vegetarian and Vegan cooking classes.

If you're interested in either, or both of these multi-session cooking courses - please send me an email with the words – Phone And Online Cooking Classes - in the subject line to: mdasNow@gmail.com.

And please, if you would be so kind, indicate in your email if you prefer the live telephone version or the live online video version of the cooking courses, and we'll let you know the dates and details when they become available.

How To Overcome Your Addictions

As promised, you will soon learn how to be victorious in overcoming the BIG PROBLEM: our actual PHYSICAL addiction to today's super-abundant calorie-rich foods.

If you've been reading straight through, or haven't taken a break lately, you may want to stand up and do a 7th inning stretch - so go ahead and stand up and stretch your arms out … and now sit down refreshed and raring to go again.

The Big Problem

In a moment you'll hear how to overcome the BIG PROBLEM: our PHYSICAL addiction to today's super-abundant calorie-rich, bad foods.

As part of that how-to, please allow me to first repeat a bit of my own personal food journey - as it may give you some inspiration.

In 1974 a few years after serving stateside in the military during the Vietnam war, I found myself with a very deep, deep chronic coughing-up-thick-brown-mucus-from-the-lungs condition.

A friend gave me Professor Arnold Ehret's Mucusless Diet Healing System book, where in 1922 Professor Ehret, by his own observation & experience became convinced that greens, vegetable-fruits & sweet fruits are the only really healthy, non-mucus causing foods, or mucus-less foods.

By following his instructions my chronic lung problem was cured.

I had immediately given up meat, chicken & eggs; and on July 4, 1976 - gave up fish.

I continued to consume a small amount of dairy products, about 2 cups per month, because I knew that India civilization had survived for millenniums on a lacto-vegetarian diet, lacto meaning milk.

27 years later in 2003 I gave up dairy when I simultaneously learned the complete story of vitamin B12 & became fully aware of the level of cruelty being done to commercial dairy cows on factory farms. Soon after that, the book *The China Study* came out & established the cancer tumor-promoting problems of dairy protein.

Finishing my personal story: In the spring of 2009 I gave up eating too much wheat – a borderline nutrient food, which cured a mild stomach acid problem I'd been having lately. And gave up oil and nuts on July 4, 2010 just like I did with fish on July 4, 1976.

I'm real patriotic.

If I knew then what I know now, I would have given up everything - all animal products, all oil and all processed foods (and in my case all nuts) - all at once in 1976. You may not have to give up nuts. **Go by your blood tests!**

My story, including giving up various legal and illegal drugs, is a story of "full stop" - versus continued addiction.

Is there anyone reading this who has quit smoking cigarettes by continuing to smoke cigarettes in moderation?

Many cheating vested interests say moderation is the key to success - but how many cigarettes is a moderate amount?

Or in the extreme case – and I'm not making a comment on WWII, I'm only using it as an example of an extreme case – how many cities destroyed by nuclear bombs is a moderate amount?

The point is: **If it's bad – zero amount is the only acceptable amount.**

Remember the director of the **USDA Energy Metabolism Laboratory**'s statement: "The most identifiable thing about the foods people **crave** is that they are highly dense in calories."

Crave Means Addicted

Well in typical vested interest ignorance - ignorance means to ignore – the director of the USDA Energy Metabolism Laboratory goes on to say that people attempting to lose weight and maintain weight loss, may benefit from advice to: "<u>accept that food cravings may not decrease in frequency</u>."

Well duh, of course cravings won't decrease in frequency if you're still "moderately" eating the highly addictive heavy foods.

That's because the USDA and so many other vested interests like: the processed food industry, the pharmaceutical industry, the medical industry including many doctors – not all, the government as a regulator, the government as a large land owner, large private land owners, lobbyists on Capitol Hill, the advertising industry and HMO's; they're all saying or at least acquiescing to:

"Moderation is the key, moderation is the key - keep on eating addictive foods. By you're continued addiction - that's how we make our living - at the cost of others, at the cost of your health & well-being and even at the cost of innocent children."

Don't Fall For It

Please, don't fall for it. You're better than that. You're NOT a sheep being lead to slaughter.

Please know that moderation is NOT the key. Zero is the key. Zero bad - Plenty good.

Because rich foods are absolutely, without a doubt, physically addictive - we are designed that way by nature – the only happy solution is to all-the-way t-total.

Like it or not at first glance – that's what it is.

Calorie rich, addictive foods are somewhat similar to nicotine or crack cocaine. Our predilection for addiction to calorie heavy foods had to be - for survival. But not now, not in the modern developed world - due to super availability and abundance.

Physical addiction is bad enough by itself, but then add to that: false food groups, false shaky pyramid schemes, wobbly-cracked spinning plates, false instructions of moderation, and false claims of starvation - all conspiring to keep you from realizing the simple and effective solution: **Eat the good foods & don't eat any of the bad foods - zero.**

It may be a temporary inconvenience - but zero bad is the only **permanent** solution.

And the permanent solution is the only easy solution – otherwise you suffer over & over & over again.

Taste Sensations

And you won't believe what - with minimal effort - what **taste sensations** await you when you break with the old narrow ways and begin to discover new foods and new combinations of foods that were there in front of you all the time, but you just didn't see – had never experienced.

It's best to eat from the beginning of the plant life cycle, from the leaf to the flower, to the fruit, to the tuber, to the legume & and don't eat any – zero – animal foods or processed foods.

Science has clearly proven this and I'll tell you more about the landmark Cornell, Oxford, China Study in a moment - but for now just understand that vested interests have conspired, consciously or unconsciously to confuse you and deny you the truth.

The calorie normal, nutrient rich and healing **Plant Life Cycle Diet** is the greatest gift.

Three Instructions Only

Now to succeed in breaking your and everyone's big problem – the addiction problem, we need rules, boundaries and limitations. That's how you maintain a healthy life.

Has anyone ever seen the Dog Whisperer?

If you have, you have seen how setting rules, boundaries and limitations on addicted dogs is totally effective. We're not doggies, but "bow, wow" - it works the same way in humans.

Drum roll please. Give me a drum roll…

Simple Rule #1) for breaking food addiction & there are only 3 rules. You may write these on a 3" x 5" card or piece of paper and **attach it to your refrigerator:**

Rule #1) Don't Buy It - Buying is eating. Buying is eating. Write it right now yourself on a 3" x 5" card (or on whatever), and in a moment when you have all three rules written down, post it on your refrigerator.

Write it down now – I'll wait right here for you:

Rule #1) Don't Buy It - Buying is eating.

I used to go to the store and buy five types of green vegetables and fruits and one "treat".

Guess what I ate **all of** as soon as I got home?

No buying and eating any unhealthy foods! **Zero**. Home or out. If you're out and someone's treating, still take only the healthy foods available.

It may be tough at first and you might fall down under pressure to choose things quickly, but in no time if you are **committed to breaking addiction** you'll become expert in knowing what to accept.

My wife and I go over this in our multi-session cooking courses. Email mdasNow@gmail.com.

Rule # 2) In the beginning, or in tough situations, don't preach to opposition.

Be cheerful and stupid. You might tell everyone - for example - that you're allergic to whatever it is – they'll usually give you a pass. If they ask for specifics, you can tell them it upsets your stomach – they can't argue with that. If they give their remedy, say, "Thanks, I'll check it out".

Even be careful in the beginning, not to come-on too strong with those who express interest in what you're doing – to much force, and they'll think you're some kind of a nut. It's not OK for others to think you're a crazy nut.

Kindly ask **friends and family** to please tolerate your apparent quirky behavior. They could be your biggest obstacles to success.

Ask for their kind help in keeping you on track - and over time, they'll see your success, and may naturally want to emulate you.

Rule # 3) Prefer to eat foods in the order of the plant LIFE CYCLE - and zero animal and any kind of processed food - zero.

Remember the Plant Life Cycle - and that the leaf is the healthiest food, followed by the bud/ flower – like broccoli, then the vegetable-fruit & sweet fruits, then the root because that's where the root fits in according to calorie heaviness and approximate harvest time, then legumes, and finally in a borderline position - whole grains. And zero animal food and any kind of processed food - ever.

Real and honest healthy eating is like a coin.

A coin has two sides. To eat healthy foods is one side of the coin, **but just as important is the other side of the coin – not to eat any, ZERO un-healthy animal foods and processed foods**.

Animal-food proponents are especially vested and don't want you to stop – it's their whole identity, it's the whole identity of modern western civilization – REALLY!

****

Animal Protein Is At Least As Bad As Animal Fat

In January 2005 the landmark study: The Cornell, Oxford, China Study was published showing that animal product intake including fish, is directly proportional to the occurrence of heart attack, cancer, stroke, Alzheimer's disease, diabetes, etc, i.e. - all the degenerative diseases of industrialization.

It's generally known that animal fat is disease-causing bad food; but the Cornell, Oxford,

China Study, the brick that broke the camel's back, established, along with many other studies - that animal protein is just as bad as animal fat. Animal protein is just as bad as animal fat.

Yes, I said it twice. Both parts are bad separately and together. In other words, all animal food is bad.

Just because we **can** eat something doesn't automatically mean, that everything we eat is good for us. Just because you **can** do something doesn't mean it's good for you. That's why there are rules, boundaries & limitations in life.

Hey, but what about fish? Isn't fish good for you... No!

According to the: **Journal of Nutrition November 2003 -** Diet, Cancer & Health Study:

"Fish intake is positively associated with breast cancer incidence rate."

The overridingly significant thing here is that this is the first large *HUMAN* study ever done directly about fish and cancer.

Eating fish is only "healthy" or "good" COMPARED to eating red meat - which is worse - but saying that fish is good for you is like saying that smoking a low-tar cigarette is good for you.

Only in comparison – but not even then.

The web address for you to read the short abstract of the fish study is:

http://www.MadhavaDas.com/fishandcancer.gif

But fear not, all is well - all is not doom and gloom because, when you give up <u>one</u> food you'll find that somehow-or-other you'll come up with at least <u>two</u> or more, sometimes many more, much healthier foods to eat and relish for their new and satisfying tastes.

As you begin or continue, your high nutrient per calorie, cardio-vascular disease reversing and anti-aging, calorie normal **Eat Your Way To Health**, **Plant Life Cycle Diet** career, if you need help finding out new foods - call me at 808-878-6821 and I'll personally tell you some.

It's not boring. Attend one of our live teleseminar or live online videoseminar cooking courses, or go all the way and attend a weekend retreat or even a multi-day boot camp - and you'll quickly see, err... taste.

The Third Need Of An Ideal Diet

Another topic and maybe a bottom line important one is that: There are 3 needs of an ideal diet.

We've covered the first need – whole, calorie normal colorful plant parts.

The second need is to fill our stomach. And by good fortune it turns out that the foods that have the highest aggregate nutrients per calorie, also have the highest volume per calorie (and per gram) and really fill your stomach.

What is the third need? Let's do another quiz – what is your answer to this question…

Variety is the what of life? _____

Because of the search for spices the world is as it is today.

European Royalty loved their eating, and they were eager to find the shortest route to India

to get the variety of spices that are – well...
the spice of life.

The phrase "Spice of Life" turns out to be a
very important phrase.

Flavorful green leaf herbs are way higher in
nutrients per calorie ratio than even the main-
course green leaf and bud-vegetables like
spinach, kale, collard and broccoli, etc. -
which along with fruits including vegetable-
fruits like green beans, sweet snap peas,
cucumbers, zucchini, eggplant, okra et cetera
are staples in the Forever The Rainbow, Eat
Your Way To Health **Plant Life Cycle Diet.**

What are some high anti-oxidant green leaf herbs?

Basil	*Marjoram*
Oregano	*Lemon Leaf*
Mint	*Lemon Grass*
Cilantro	*Savory*
Dill	*Tarragon*
Bay Leaf	*Indian Curry Leaf*

And the are you going to Scarburofair spices:
Parsley, Sage, Rosemary & Thyme

Before the year 1900 these herbs and other spices and flavorings were widely used... now its - sugar, salt and fat.

After the turn of the 20th century, Mr. Wesson figured out how to make a fortune out of discarded old cottonseeds – and the race was on.

And then in the bogus USDA food groups pyramid - oil even became a so-called "food group". At least the new cracked plate doesn't have that.

Today herbs and other spices & flavorings are still easily available. You can buy them in larger sizes in wholesale stores. (Be sure to use them and don't let them petrify like my dear sister did.)

The flavor in herbs and spices, and the dark color pigments in plants are synonymous with anti-oxidants.

Resveritrol is found naturally in the skin of dark whole grapes. We should all eat whole dark grapes.

Recap

As stated in *The Pleasure Trap,* Elvis Presley's life is a metaphor for our BIG Problem of today: physical addiction to super-abundant, super-rich foods and drugs that almost no business and possibly most of your relatives don't want you to stop eating or taking.

Our addiction to super-abundant, super-rich, cheap calorie-heavy foods, and drugs is not beneficial for us.

Vested interests don't want you to quit.

Calorie Restriction = Calorie Normality.

Nutrient Density = Nutrients per calorie, not per gram.

Greens, vegetable-fruits, fruits and other whole plant parts are the best things for you - not food groups, pyramids, plates, medical procedures, animal products, oil, sugar or drugs.

Only **total** self-control breaks addiction. Only teetotaling will cure your ills.

Trade in "Drugs and surgery" medicine for "Never get sick in the first place" food medicine.

There's a whole new world of cooking & spicing for you to discover - a whole new world of **taste sensations**.

There's a whole new world of vibrant health, a cleanness and lightness of mind, body and spirit awaiting your call. All you have to do is believe… And take action.

Beauty Is Master

My philosophical and spiritual mentor, B.R. Shridhar says, "Beauty is master. All are searching for beauty. Truth is beauty. Love is beauty."

To act in accord with the laws of nature is also beauty - or at least it keeps us out of trouble.

Most of us would like to avoid sickness, and delay the event called death. If you are in this group, the Eat Your Way To Health **Plant Life Cycle Diet** is for you.

In a world governed by the law of action and reaction, also known as karma, if you pull and release a rubber band it snaps back; if you smoke cigarettes and don't eat fruits and vegetables you get lung cancer;

if you eat low nutrient per calorie animal and processed foods your cells age faster, you get diseased, and you may pile up weight over time. That's the science.

Trust And The Fish

I once worked at a mountain reservoir that had an overflow stream. There was a drought and the overflow stream dried up into separate pools. After a day or two I noticed a big fish was trapped in one of the pools. I knew he would soon use all of the oxygen in the water so I decided to scoop him up in a bucket and take him up and put him in the large reservoir.

But whenever I would approach him with the bucket - break the water surface with the bucket - he would swim away in fear. Since I didn't do much at the reservoir except mostly watch the leaves fall off the trees, I decided to take another approach.

I very, very gradually put my hand in the water and over a period of about an hour-and-a-half to two hours I slowly, slowly shuffled along the bank and moved my hand closer and closer to that fish until finally I could touch him.

And then he actually let me hold him in the palm of my hand and I slid him over and put him in the bucket and took him up and put him in the reservoir. As he swam away, it looked like he turned and lifted one fin as if to say, "Thanks man."

The Same Conclusion

The Eat Your Way To Health, **Plant Life Cycle Diet** is a health, longevity, weight loss, and kindness diet based on scientific research. Ancient humans also had their Fountain of Youth, No Hunger, Calorie Normal **Plant Life Cycle Diet**.

They didn't have modern science or use the scientific method, but somehow they reached the same conclusion and they wrote it down in their Holy Books. Or God did.

Maybe there was a time, or even now there is a place, where everyone communicates on an **affectionate** personal level with each other, regardless of bodily covering whether it be racial, ethnic, national, religious or **interspecies**.

Epilogue And Summary

Dr. Robert Vogel of the University of Maryland Medical Center and professor of medicine and director of clinical vascular biology at the University of Maryland School of Medicine has performed - as others following in his footsteps have - many of what is called the Brachial Artery Tourniquet Test.

Several groups of test subjects have the brachial artery in their arm measured by a sonogram.

After eating various meals of meat, fish, eggs, dairy, fried foods, and salad with added oil including olive oil - or after eating meals of whole, calorie normal plant parts; and after a tourniquet has stopped all blood flow to their lower arm for 5 minutes, each test subject's brachial artery is again measured.

After a **fruit and vegetable** meal when the tourniquet is released the subject's brachial artery springs back to life and DILATES to a size larger than the original sonogram showed, allowing great quantities of fresh oxygenated blood to flow.

Guess what happens to the arteries of the animal and oil eaters?

Ahhh… nothing. The artery barely allows <u>any</u> blood to flow when it is desperately needed.

This is why lots of people feel chest pain or suddenly drop dead when doing labor like shoveling snow or even mild labor like climbing up stairs. The heart needs extra blood but their oil and animal ravaged coronary (like a crown) arteries that surround their heart FAIL TO DIALATE.

Quick Fix

Here's how to look & feel up to 10 years younger in only 3 days:

Over a span of just 3 days eat on a daily basis only four measured packed cups of lightly cooked and spiced green leafy vegetables per day, and one cup of dark colored berries per day. Greens may be blended.

You will be assured of getting all the nutrients you need for that time period almost without calories. You'll reverse 10 years of biological aging - and FEEL 10 years younger in only a few days.

Then CONTINUE to eat a greens and other vegetables and fruits staple diet including tubers, some legumes, and possibly some grains, with <u>zero</u> animal, oil, and junk foods -

for lifelong maximum health, vitality, good looks and longevity.

Don't be cowed down by the economic and face-saving desires of vested interests - including relatives - into disrespecting your own self.

The benefits of the **Plant Life Cycle Diet** are great - maximum life span and vigorous health, along with good looks; and it's never too late to begin.

You have already made a great start by reading this book.

Now I challenge each and every one of you to put your money where your mouth is, and to actually start eating those green leaf $100 bills and other healthy whole plant parts.

We know you are serious about your health, so you are invited to join my wife Sunanda and I for a weekend or longer of hands-on eating fun and talks.

Please email Madhava and Sunanda to make arrangements.

mdasNow@gmail.com

Two Page Summery Of Entire Book

• Animal foods and processed foods are unhealthy.

• A diet of a variety of whole plant foods is healthy and totally satisfying.

• From a CR/CN perspective the highest-nutrient-density-per-calorie whole plant foods are the healthiest.

• Nutrient density for all practical purposes follows the plant's reproductive life cycle - descending in order from edible leaf and stem, through bud, flower, fruit, tuber/root and seed as calorie density increases.

• Practically speaking a diet of any reasonable combination of whole plant parts, which does not exceed normal average historical calorie intake levels of human animals living in a natural environment, is healthy.

• What is called calorie restriction in humans is actually pre-industrial calorie normality. A varied and filling whole plant life cycle food diet automatically leads to calorie normality without counting calories or artificially restricting calorie intake.

• Persons following a healthy whole plant-food diet with weight problems or with high blood-cholesterol levels above 150 total & 80 LDL, may adjust their eating to include more of the calorie-light green leafy and other vegetables and fruits, and less of the more calorie dense, peas, beans, whole grains, seeds and other high fat plant foods.

Too much dried fruit or fruit juice, both of which are slightly processed/fractionated foods, and both of which have high calorie density (we shouldn't really be eating any of these) can also cause weight problems and too-high blood-fat levels.

If despite minimizing nut intake, your total and LDL blood cholesterol levels remain above 150 and 80 mg/dL respectively, then for degenerative disease proofing's sake you may eliminate nut intake – not because there is anything wrong with nuts but because in your particular case you cannot tolerate the slightly higher calorie density that including a few nuts in your diet affords you.

In other words, eliminate the calorie densest foods one by one from your diet until your blood cholesterol consistently stays below 150 and 80! No need to count calories.

• The plant's life cycle explains healthy eating.

• Adopt the **PLANT LIFE CYCLE DIET** for superior health, kindness and cognizant, vibrant long life.

• <u>**KNOW**</u> **& CONTROL your cholesterol numbers.**

Only The Best

You will see thousands and thousands of references from apparent authorities to eat cancer promoting chicken and fish for example, because they have lower or "better" fat than red meats. And to eat olive oil and other coronary blood vessel attacking processed oils, because they supposedly have good fats. And you will read various other recommendations contrary to what you have read here, including about blood cholesterol and about so many other things.

Don't listen to them. They are spouting half-truth or are just plain wrong - well-intentioned maybe – but wrong none-the-less.

We are talking about the best – they are giving popular second best. If you want second best that's your choice. But I don't think you do because you have happily finished reading this book.

Maybe you will fall down once in a while – we all do – but don't give up. Just brush yourself off and get back to the valiant effort to be the **best** you can be.

You can do it. And you will take great joy from it because you are sincere, committed, and surrendered.

Final Words On
Health And Kindness

The young people of today are to be commended for ethically refusing to connect themselves with animal slaughter and cruelty.

Older persons who give up animal products and processed foods for health reasons are very smart and are also to be commended.

For whatever reasons you have read this book, you are to be commended.

And now the promised final quote:

"I've always felt that animals are the purest spirits in the world. They don't fake or hide their feelings, and they are the most loyal creatures on Earth. And somehow we humans think we're smarter—what a joke." ~ Pink

Key Word And Phrase Index

About the Author:

Madhava Das, also known as "Dasa", is president of Nutritional Research Maui & holds a Cornell University Certificate in Plant-based Nutrition.

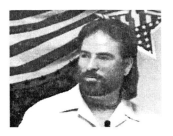

Before taking to healthy living, Dasa, as a young man suffered from chronic lung congestion and extremely high blood pressure.

In 1975 Madhava received professor Arnold Ehret's Mucusless Diet Healing System Lessen Course completed in 1922 which says vegetables and fruits are mucusless foods - similar to the modern research based Calorie Normal, **Plant Life Cycle Diet**; and in 1976 adopted Ehret's diet, more or less on faith, as science had not yet fully discovered and established the health benefits of the high nutrient per calorie, calorie normal, whole-food plant-based diet.

Dasa is also a pioneering aviator being an original founder of the modern sport of hang gliding and the United States Hang Gliding Association; and having contributed to the design of the first successful human powered aircraft, the Gossamer Condor, now hanging at the Smithsonian Air & Space Museum in

Washington, D.C. beside the original Wright Brothers Flyer and the Apollo 11 command module, Columbia, that took the first humans to walk on the moon.

Madhava may be contacted at:
mdasNow@gmail.com or mdasa1@gmail.com
